D1291260

Body, Mind, and Mouth

Life's Eating Connection

Margaret Marshall

abbott press®
A DIVISION OF WRITER'S DIGEST

Body, Mind, and Mouth
Life's Eating Connection

Copyright © 2012 Margaret Marshall

All rights reserved. No part of this book may be used or reproduced by any means, graphic, electronic, or mechanical, including photocopying, recording, taping or by any information storage retrieval system without the written permission of the publisher except in the case of brief quotations embodied in critical articles and reviews.

ISBN: 978-1-4582-0680-0 (sc)
ISBN: 978-1-4582-0679-4 (hc)
ISBN: 978-1-4582-0678-7 (e)

Library of Congress Control Number: 2012921145

Abbott Press books may be ordered through booksellers or by contacting:

Abbott Press
1663 Liberty Drive
Bloomington, IN 47403
www.abbottpress.com
Phone: 1-866-697-5310

Because of the dynamic nature of the Internet, any web addresses or links contained in this book may have changed since publication and may no longer be valid. The views expressed in this work are solely those of the author and do not necessarily reflect the views of the publisher, and the publisher hereby disclaims any responsibility for them.

Any people depicted in stock imagery provided by Thinkstock are models, and such images are being used for illustrative purposes only.

Certain stock imagery © Thinkstock.

Printed in the United States of America

Abbott Press rev. date: 11/30/2012

"When you eat well, you live well. When you eat healthy, you are healthy. When you nourish your body, you nourish your mind."

—Margaret Marshall

Contents

Foreword . . . . *xi*

Introduction . . . . *xiii*

Eat Anything, Not Everything 1

Three Magic Words 9

What's in It for You? 21

Your Inner Dialogue 31

Eat What You Like; Learn How to Eat It 39

And…Action! 51

Find the Time 61

Now, the Science 75

The 10-Step WEIGH to a Healthy Body 79

Cooking Tips for Lower-Calorie Cooking 83

Let's Go Out to Eat 85

Epilogue *87*

Foreword

I have been a client of Margaret Marshall for a number of years. She is a talented life coach, teaching life's lessons with intelligence, charm, and caring. Her advice and ideas are always upbeat, emphasizing that you must care about your inner self, your health, and your well-being in order to properly care for yourself and for others. She gives you the knowledge you need to do this, encourages you to practice new skills, and advises patience in achieving your goals. What others might perceive as a setback, Margaret regards as simply an opportunity to turn a situation into a positive learning experience.

Margaret is a warm caring woman, whose qualities shine through in these pages, just as they do when you are face-to-face with her. With this book, you have the next best thing to having her beside you on your journey to a healthier life. What she offers is not an eating plan, but a life plan. You just know that she is in your corner, cheering you on in your efforts to improve your health and your life!

Judith Lee Hallock, Ph.D.

Introduction

"There is always a choice, and each time, you'll get what you choose."
—Margaret Marshall

Are you, your friends, co-workers, or family members overweight? Is it affecting attitude, productivity, level of joy, and success? Imagine how a shift in thought and a change of eating patterns would affect your level of success, joy, motivation, and direction in your life! Envision goals once believed out of reach to be possible. You can make one of the most difficult things (sustained weight loss/weight management) easier. Picture how improved your life would be if you restructured, recreated, and reignited your eating satisfaction. You would achieve your ideal body weight, optimum health, and entry into that "thinner world" that you previously thought only others could achieve.

I offer you the story of my weight issues, struggles, insights, and victories from which I have learned a great deal, as well as the experiences and stories of my clients from which I have also learned a lot. I have structured my life and surroundings to manage my weight and maintain a healthy body size. I am five-feet, seven-inches tall and a size ten. From time to time, the number on the scale changes minimally. However, my goal remains the size ten.

I was an overweight child, the only girl in a family with four brothers. My father, with his military background and heavy himself, would say to me, "Margaret, we will fight the battle of the bulge together." My brothers, who were thin, nicknamed me "Margaret, Margaret, the big fat target!" My mother told me stories about when she was young. She said she was so skinny that the nuns sent her home for lunch each day so she could eat potatoes and drink milk shakes.

Why me? Why was my mother sent home to have milk shakes, while I couldn't even enjoy a dish of ice cream without being told that it was not good for me? Why was I larger than my older brother? Needless to say, these and other experiences formed the body image/self-image that would follow me always.

My maternal grandmother passed away from colon cancer when she was fifty-two, and I was three. I have no memory of her, although I was also named after her. My mother often told me that I reminded her of her mother. I always felt a connection to my grandmother and have seen photographs of her taken throughout her life. One was her wedding picture. She was a tall, beautiful bride, standing proudly in her wedding gown next to her handsome groom. I was often told, "You are tall like your grandmother." (My mother and father were not tall.) I also saw pictures of her near the end of her life. She still appeared tall, but she also looked heavy. I believed my future would bring the same fate.

Throughout my teens, I went on crazy diets that might sound familiar: the cabbage diet, the yogurt diet, and the starvation diet (to name a few). While looking through old family photographs, I noticed that I would only pose for a picture if I liked the way I looked, which was most likely after a fad diet or starving myself for days. My twenties brought my marriage to Chris, and we had two children, Megan and Michael. My marriage and the birth of both children were body altering. By the time I was thirty, I was a size 16, totally out of control with my eating, and wondering what my future body weight would be. I was overweight, frumpy, and miserable!

At age thirty and a size 16, I began to disconnect with people. I hated to have repairmen in the house, and I detested going to business functions with Chris. It was not about the way I looked, it was about the way I felt. I wondered what size I would be at age fifty. But, of course, the real question was, did I want to spend my adult life in an over-weight, unhealthy body? After all, I had been told that I was like my grandmother in many ways, and history can repeat itself.

When I was thirty, I reluctantly joined the local WeightWatchers® group, thinking, "OK, I've tried everything else, now I'll try this." Well, I took control of my eating, my weight, and myself. By thirty-one, I was a size 10.

Shortly after, I began working for WeightWatchers® as a group leader and kept that position for seventeen years. Early on, I realized you couldn't get your power from a commercial diet program; the power must come from within you. I realized people joined and continually rejoined diet programs many times over because they had never believed in themselves or in their own power. For my own well-being and lifestyle, I developed my own philosophies that enriched me and enabled me to continue living my life in the size 10 that was so important to me.

Instinctively, I knew sustained weight loss is more than counting calories, and collecting new recipes. Questions similar to, "What kind of cheese should I eat...fat-free or part-skim?" or "What's the best popcorn?" became increasingly wearisome to me.

When my youngest son left for college, my role as a mother was redefined. I resigned from WeightWatchers® to follow my passion to work with people on an individual basis, empowering them to discover their issues, barriers, and challenges, and enabling them to break through them. In September of 2004, I established Margaret Marshall Assoc., Inc., and the Why Weight coaching method to implement my mission: discovering the body, mind, and mouth connection in each individual life. The body, mind, and mouth connection is the realization of how your mouth (your eating), whether consciously or not, relates and reacts to the health of your body, your mind, and outside stimuli.

My expertise is that of a speaker, a weight loss/wellness coach, and a realist. I have the knowledge and ability to guide individuals to a healthy mindset and lifestyle. I work to empower others to structure their lives and circumstances while educating them to make decisions in their best interests. I'm happy to report that today we are flourishing, with clients in several states and locales. We have been featured on television and radio, as well as in magazines and newspapers. I have been recognized as a contributing expert in the field of weight loss and weight control. I conduct seminars and workshops, and give keynote addresses on various topics related to health and wellness with a focus on weight control.

A healthy body and mind is essential to people of all ages. Healthy eating and a basic understanding of good nutrition are vital at every age. My clients range from high-school students to seniors. Depending on our stage of life, we eat and respond to situations differently. My clients include clergy, educators, executives and blue collar workers, firemen and police officers, medical doctors, therapists, addiction counselors, psychiatrists, attorneys, expectant and nursing mothers, young parents, and grandparents.

I've helped people through illnesses and guided people with their eating patterns as they went through radiation or chemotherapy, where nourishing your body must be the focus. I've helped people eat to improve or reverse effects of food allergies, diabetes, high cholesterol, high blood pressure, and celiac disease. I've worked with anorexic women who wish to conceive and start their family. These women have done damage to their bodies over the years, and fertility doctors require them to be a certain body weight before treatment. My focus is to help them eat healthfully to *gain weight* and gain strength in order to conceive. I've worked with caregivers to help them to take the time to care for themselves as well as their loved one. My clients have included retired people whose time is no longer structured so their eating suffers. Their eating patterns and schedules changed after they became full-time babysitters for their grandchildren or even found themselves raising grandchildren. I've worked with individuals or families who are grief stricken over the death of a loved one. At first, they generally don't feel like eating due to grief, but they make themselves eat to preserve their strength; over time, food becomes their comfort. Body weight and eating are intimate topics. They affect us all, yet there is a great need for individual attention.

For the most part, I guide overweight individuals to eliminate destructive eating patterns. Some patterns are inherited from previous generations and are deeply seated in traditions and ethnicity, while some are learned by current conditions and environment.

I encourage clients to practice new, productive eating patterns, while respecting the value systems of their heritage. With my help, they are able to create a lifestyle that produces ideal body weight, good health, and inner peace.

A very dear friend told me, "Your grandmother did shape you; she gave you passion and direction in your life." She and others helped me to realize my own connection between my body, my mind, and my mouth.

Stepping away from the constraints of the commercial program allowed me to think and strategize, as well as further study eating habits and people's responses to different situations. This transformation has been liberating. I pass that knowledge on to my clients and to participants at my seminars, workshops, and keynote addresses.

Through experience and example, I teach the concepts of weight loss without drugs, surgery, or tasteless diet products. There is no magic to weight loss. You must eat healthily, eat the correct balance of food for your body, and move. You need to master successful skills and habits by practicing. You don't need gimmicks or weight-loss products. You need information, education, and direction. Knowledge, practice, and patience are the cornerstone to managing body weight.

You already know there are many ways to lose weight. This book is not about quick ways to shed pounds or "revolutionary" new treatments that soon become obsolete. Rather, it's proven strategies, thoughts, ideas, and scenarios to help you lead a thin healthy life, *throughout your life*. It is a guide on mindsets that enable you to live in a thin, healthy body. My objective is to shorten your learning curve and help you enjoy your body for many years to come. You will begin to understand that weight loss at any cost is not good weight loss. A rapid loss is not lasting, and leads to an overweight existence throughout your life.

First, create relationships and a lifestyle that work for *you*, and then concentrate on good nutrition. This book guides you to gain control of your thoughts, feelings, actions, environment, and body. Your thinking dictates your feelings and your feelings dictate your eating. Concentrate on your thinking.

Regardless of your age, occupation, or position in life, this book is dedicated to encouraging you to make daily choices and constructive actions consistent with the direction and results you desire. Begin to appreciate good health. Allow yourself to live with inner peace regardless of the stresses in your life. When you take good care of your body and really embrace it, the feeling from within will trump outside stresses. However, you must hold on tightly. Life's twists and turns sometimes have a way of winning. The key is, don't give up!

By eating well, exercising, and always caring for your body, you can improve your life in many ways.

» **Blood Pressure, High Cholesterol, and Diabetes:** Although these diseases or conditions have a great deal to do with aging or genetics, how you eat and your body size play an enormous role in managing—or avoiding—these conditions all together.

» **Fatigue:** Carrying excess body weight is taxing on your body. Take a ten-pound bag of potatoes and carry it all day. Witness how tired it makes you. Carrying excess weight every day, in everything you do, is exhausting!

» **Depression:** How you feel on the inside shows on the outside. If you are not feeling positive about yourself, you internalize your reactions to outside stimuli in a negative manner leading to depression. Having said that, I have met many overweight individuals who have claimed, "Regardless of my size, I'm happy." That's fabulous, but I wonder why they need to say, "Regardless of my size...?" What's not being said?

» **Chronic pain:** Excess weight wreaks havoc on joints. For example, every pound on your body puts six pounds of pressure on your knees. If you're thirty pounds overweight, that's 180 pounds of additional pressure on your knees.

» **Mental attitude and sex drive:** Both are closely related. Only you know what your mental attitude is and how it manifests in areas of your life. When your body weight affects your mental attitude, leaving you feeling that you are less than you are, how can it not affect your sex drive?

» **Your respect for others and your ability to love others:** When self-respect and self-love are lost, your ability to show others how much you love and respect them is diminished. Your weight should play no part in self-respect or self-love, but your self-care does. No matter how much you weigh, hold on to self-care and you will keep your self-respect and self-love.

Your weight and health will not immediately change, but your outlook and attitude can, and that will be the start of changing your weight and health.

The weight-loss industry is a $60-billion industry. Believe me when I say there is nothing new. I offer you my perspective and my experience of a lifetime of managing my weight. I have made it my life's work and passion to help others. I have worked with nearly 10,000 people. Many times, I have witnessed firsthand the power you have when you believe in yourself. I offer you realistic steps to overcome the stresses in your life as you care for yourself.

This is the story of my journey of education, experience, and discovery, as well as the stories of my family, friends, and clients. I want to inspire you as these people have inspired me. There is no need to waste years gaining and losing weight. I challenge you to change your mindset and eating patterns now. You can achieve your ideal body weight, and live healthfully and happily.

You might see yourself, your feelings, and your habits in these stories. When you do, recognize you are not alone. Reading the stories will help you understand your own behaviors and give you insight to a different or more efficient approach, which leads to new and exhilarating results.

Earlier in my life, I was not motivated by the goal of good health. Now that I am in my fifties, I am! My plan is to enter the future decades of my life healthy and medication-free. I wish you the same future.

Eat Anything, Not Everything

"Tell me what you eat, and I shall tell you what you are."
—Jean-Anthelme Brillat-Savarin (1755-1826)
Author: "The Physiology of Taste", Published 1825

You are *not* overweight because you eat. You are overweight because you overeat. There is a fine line between eating and overeating, but it could be difficult to discern because of your relationship with food.

Is food a friend or foe? Do you reward or punish yourself with food, or do you allow food to nourish your body and nurture your soul? Think about what food really means to you, the eating habits you have, how they were created, and where they are leading you. Food is meant to nourish your body and keep you healthy. Many of the foods we eat neither nourish us nor keep us healthy. They are full of artificial ingredients, coloring, chemicals, sugar, fat, and sodium. People put these ingredients into their bodies every day. These ingredients wreak havoc on your health and internal organs. The resulting excess body fat and ill health could show up during your lifetime.

When babies are born, parents are instructed to feed them every three to four hours. They are never told: "Give them a bottle when they feel happy or sad. When they are bored, feed them. If someone is mistreating them, offer them a bottle. Always give them one when they are watching television. Then, every time you take them to the movies, super-size their bottle." Babies cry when they are hungry or when they are wet. If they are crying because they are wet and are offered a bottle, they spit it out with dissatisfaction.

Look at the animal kingdom. They eat on instinct. Put soda in your dog's water dish and see what happens. He won't touch it! When your dog is tired, he doesn't eat, he sleeps.

On the other hand, we are taught to eat for any reason and every occasion. We no longer know what true hunger feels like, and we are afraid of it. Our bodies have been designed to eat every three to four hours throughout our lives, and we condition them to eat more often.

On a recent cruise, I was sitting on deck near the buffet waiting for Chris to arrive to have breakfast together. A mother and young daughter of about three or four were sitting near me. I overheard the mother speaking with her daughter. She told the little girl that she must attend the children's camp today. The little girl began to cry, and she said she didn't want to go. The mother explained that Mommy and Daddy needed adult time, so she was going to have kid time today. The little girl continued wailing that she didn't want to go. Finally the mother said, "After Daddy and I pick you up this afternoon, we'll get ice cream." Bingo! The tears immediately stopped and the little girl told her mom what flavor she wanted. This tiny little person had already learned food and treats are the answers and rewards.

Food should be your friend, but somewhere between our first days and our last days we learn to abuse food and, in turn, abuse our bodies.

There should never be a food that is off limits, but there should be limits on food. If you are eating foods that bring down your mood and destroy your health, you are abusing your body with food. If you eat foods that nourish your body, they will nurture your soul and mind, making you a happier and healthier person at any weight.

In any daily situation, function, or party, rate the foods offered from one to ten, ten being the foods you love most, regardless of what they are.

Eat your eights, nines and tens. Leave out foods that are mediocre! Don't waste your time or calories on them.

For example, I love ice cream. What I've learned is I don't love all ice creams. Some flavors are a ten, while others are a four or five rating. Non-fat or low-fat ice creams are a three or four and frankly not worth my time. When I truly want ice cream, I go out to a local ice-cream parlor, order a serving of a flavor that I rate a ten with a topping that's also a ten! Then, I sit down and enjoy every bite. Now, if I did this every day, I would gain weight. However, ice cream is a food I don't keep in my freezer. If a half-gallon of my favorite ice cream is in my freezer, odds are it will not be there at the end of the day!

Cashews are another food I don't keep in the house. I like them too much and have a hard time controlling the quantity I eat. I will eat them at a party when other people are present. You may find hard-to-control foods easier to control--and more enjoyable--in the company of others. I'm not saying you can never eat these foods, I'm just saying that you need to learn to eat them so they don't work against you.

Identify what foods you rate as an eight, nine, or ten and find ways to enjoy them. High-fat foods like cashews and ice cream will derail your weight-loss efforts if there are no limits. *Eat what you like; learn how to eat.* Make your food work for you, not against you.

A number of my clients had followed a carbohydrate-free diet. They lost weight quickly, but once they reintroduced their beloved carbohydrates, they regained their weight almost as quickly. When you eat what you like, and learn how to eat, nothing need be deleted. You will train yourself—and it can become automatic for you—to eat items at the most effective time.

Eat for a reason, not an excuse. A client told me she was taking her kids to a local amusement park. She was concerned about how she was going to eat that day. I asked her what she found so challenging about it. After some thought, she said, "It's not really that the food itself is so tempting. I just really enjoy having ice cream with my kids." That's eating for a reason. Her reason was she wanted to enjoy time and ice cream with her kids. Her excuses could have been: "I'm going to the park, where all kinds of different foods are abundant, so I'll just eat them like I always do," or "I went to the park yesterday where I blew it, so it doesn't matter what I eat today." She could have followed her past patterns of overeating. However, after she thought about her plans for the day, she realized that having ice cream together was essential to attending the park. Having excess food was not.

Excuses are everywhere. Just pick one out of the air! *Reasons* are different than excuses. Ask yourself: "What do I want most?" Be specific with your answer: Better health, less chronic pain, fewer medications, a smaller clothes size, or maybe the ability to tuck your shirt in comfortably? You have to decide. One never really knows what weight loss means to individuals and what motivates them.

Two of my clients, an officer with the New York City Police Department (NYPD) and his wife, had decided to lose weight together. They both wanted to eat better, get and feel healthier, and set a good example for their children. One evening at the start of our session, after the husband had lost about forty pounds, he exclaimed, "Now, I can close my vest securely!" I asked, "What do you mean?" He explained that after graduating from the police academy, he had been issued a bulletproof vest. Lately, because of his excess weight, he could only close his vest tightly on the right side, leaving a gap on the left side of his body. He knew that if he had ever gotten in a shootout, he would have to face right as he drew his gun. He had also been concerned that he would be passed over for a promotion due to his weight and his inability to move quickly.

On the other hand, his wife added, "Last Friday, we went to a party, and he looked HOT!" He gleamed (I had always suspected that was his motivation). What a change forty pounds made! It could have saved his life and the future of his young family. Shortly thereafter, he became a New York City detective.

Although you may never be in a position to wear a bulletproof vest, you may be able to identify with the vulnerability of having the vest open on one side. As the police officer did, we attempt to hide our vulnerabilities. Eventually, they can no longer be hidden and the weaknesses are exposed. Then, they take over, leaving us powerless, *unless* we find a way to overcome them. Find your way, take control, and close the gap.

Each of my clients is motivated by different goals. Another client told me his future plans were to open his own business. He wanted to look "presentable" to attract clients. His weight loss was part of his *business plan!* One client told me she was having trouble conceiving, and the fertility doctor would not work with her until she lost weight. Another client said she just wants to live, and worries every day will be her last due to her weight. Many clients want to decrease or delete medications that they are forced to take to counteract conditions caused by being overweight. One woman confided that she wants to be a "Hot Momma," and yet another said she wanted to be "sexified!"

Know what your "payoff" or "price tag" is on your weight loss. Your payoff is the benefit to you and how this could enhance your life. Your price tag is what it will cost you to continue destructive habits. Get a clear mental picture of both. Share the picture of your "payoff" with someone you trust, and bring it to life.

Many people claim their life's circumstances are out of their control. They say the only thing they have control over is food, and that's why they overeat. If you are overweight, you *do not* have control over food. It's quite the opposite. Food is controlling you. In reality, you are stronger than any food item, and within the next minute you *can* be in control of your food. It is a choice! As you begin controlling your food, it's amazing what other circumstances you will find yourself controlling. You will learn how to deal with other situations that seemed out of your control.

When you are challenged with particular foods, remember those foods are only what you want *now*. They are visible, tangible, and available. To counteract that, always keep in mind the picture of what you want *most*, whatever that is to you. Make it concrete. Have something close by to remind you, such as a picture of yourself or someone you admire, a small sports car you want to drive, or maybe a certain outfit. It makes no difference, as long as it's what *you* want. Unfortunately, we are a society of instant gratification. Weight loss is never instant, but if accomplished correctly, it can be very gratifying. Never give up what you want *most* for what you want *now*.

Hunger has very little to do with an overweight person's lifestyle. The chances are they have never experienced hunger. They are so anxious about feeling hungry that they'll avoid it at any cost, and the cost is enormous. The price people pay is their body, health, quality of life, and inner peace. Hunger is not the enemy; the over-stuffed feeling is! Hunger is your body telling you it's time to eat. Get comfortable with the feeling of hunger. Once you are comfortable with it, you will be better equipped to make good food choices. When you are fearful of getting hungry, you may just grab anything and eat.

If you eat nothing all day and never feel hungry, you have slowed your metabolism into a starvation mode. Starvation mode simply means your body wants to use as few calories as possible to sustain itself, because your body believes you are not nourishing it. Calories are a measurement of energy. Because your body doesn't know when you will give it more energy in the form of calories, it begins protecting itself for survival by conserving calories.

You need to eat to avoid starvation mode. True hunger means you've used most of the energy from your last meal or snack, but you haven't hit the stage yet where you are in danger of overeating. You'll burn more calories by eating throughout the day. But remember, you can eat throughout the day and still be malnourished. Always choose wisely.

You know you have had enough to eat when you feel satisfied. This takes awareness, practice, and sometimes an immediate reaction to what your body is trying to tell you. If you are eating out of momentum or habit until you're full or until you're stuffed, you are destined to be uncomfortable and overweight.

In the event your schedule does not allow you to take a break, carry a small snack with you for when you might be hungry later. A little box of raisins and some nuts can do the trick, or carry a cup of cold milk in a thermal coffee cup.

Always focus on what you are going to eat, never on what you are *not* going to eat. Tell yourself, "I'm going to have <u>strawberries</u>." *Never* say, "I won't have those <u>cookies</u>." In the latter case, your subconscious hears only "cookies" and will lead you right to them.

I can recall when I was a young mother and took Megan, Michael, and their friends to the movies. I always drove there thinking, "I'm *not* going to have Goobers (chocolate covered peanuts). During the ten-minute drive to the movie theatre, I repeated that in my head. I thought I was convincing myself not to buy any Goobers. But, each time I paid for the movie tickets, I went straight to the snack counter to get a box of Goobers, the very same treat I had just chanted against for ten minutes. Then, of course, I would get mad at myself, feel guilty and defeated, which usually led to further eating!

In reality, I was focusing on the candy, because our brains don't register words like *can't, don't,* and *won't*. For example, if you say: "I'm *not* going to have Goobers," and delete the "*not,*" as your brain would do, what you hear is: "I'm *going* to have Goobers." As an exercise right now, close your eyes, and "don't picture your bedroom." What did you see?

When I told myself *what* I was going to have instead of what I was *not* going to have, the visit to the candy counter changed effortlessly. Same scene, different words: I drove to the movie—still with a carload of excited kids—but this time, I repeated to myself, "I'm going to have a cup of coffee." When I paid for the tickets and took the kids to the snack counter, I ordered a cup of coffee because I had focused on what I was going to have, the coffee.

Most of us can multi-task, but we can only think one thought at a time. Think about your relationship with food. Gaining weight is a thoughtless, mindless pattern. As you eat—and especially overeat—your thoughts are usually on other things. Weight loss and weight management takes thought. When you think and plan what to eat and when to eat, you are in command.

Your thoughts control your eating and your weight. It's the body, mind, and mouth connection.

Points to Remember

- You are overweight because you overeat.
- You may find hard-to-control foods easier to control in the company of others.
- Weight loss is never instant, but done correctly is very gratifying.
- Always focus on what you are going to eat, and plan foods you look forward to eating.

Three Magic Words

You have to expect things of yourself before you can do them.
—Michael Jordan
Professional basketball player, *1984-2003*

When I hold workshops or seminars, mostly filled with people who are not comfortable in their own skin, I ask everyone to look into an imaginary mirror and use three words to describe what they see. These people are various age groups and differing weights. I hear many words in response—all of them negative—and that's only from those who are willing to share. I wonder what words are in the minds of those not willing to share? Take a minute, and look into your own imaginary mirror. What three words describe you?

The one word I am always guaranteed to hear is *fat*. Is fat one of your words? Is fat your body image, self-image, or self-worth? I think people have different definitions of the word fat. Personally, I cringe when I hear anybody describe themselves as fat. I have a hard time saying it. When I am interviewed on television or radio, I even ask the interviewer not to use the word, "fat."

Fat is the F word to me. It's always used in a derogatory way. Once you believe yourself to be fat, it becomes your body image and/or your self-image. You embrace it and own it as a word that defines you. As long as you believe this, you will continue to see yourself as fat regardless of your weight. If you believe yourself to be *overweight,* that belief seems to change as your body weight decreases. It seems people can easily shed the overweight status in their mind, yet they never seem to let go of the fat mindset, which allows weight to return. It's a self-fulfilled prophecy.

Consider fat to be a state of feeling, not a state of being. This means you only *feel* fat. If you can grasp this major concept, you can benefit from my twenty-plus years of studying the patterns of overweight people. Now, I know all about body composition and the existence of body fat; we are not addressing that here. I'm talking about the *feeling* of being fat.

Let's imagine we have two people, Jane and Jean. They are the same height and same weight. Both weigh 250 pounds. A year ago Jane weighed 300 pounds, but she worked during the year at losing weight, so Jane feels magnificent. Fat is not a word she would use to describe herself. She may feel she has more weight to lose, but fat? No!

On the other hand, Jean spent the last year overeating and gaining weight. A year ago she weighed 200 and now weighs 250. Jean now feels fat. People like Jean say things like, "When I look at pictures of myself at 200 pounds, I think 'I thought I was fat *then!*'" It's that fat feeling, in part, that enabled Jean to continue putting on excess body weight. It's the body, mind, and mouth connection.

Both Jane and Jean had weighed exactly the same, but changed their body weight by fifty pounds. The fifty pounds up or down is the deciding factor in how they feel, define, and treat themselves.

Sometimes a client says, "I had a hard week, I feel so fat today." When they get onto the scale and discover they have lost a pound or two, the *feeling* of being fat always dissipates.

To simplify this point, I stand five-feet, seven-inches tall and most people would consider me tall. Often I feel tall, especially when I am standing with others shorter than I am. But very often I feel short, mainly when I'm in the company of taller people. My height never changes, but I know how it feels to be tall and to be short. Whether I feel short or tall always dictates how I hold myself upright.

If you feel fat, you live in that feeling, treat yourself so, and continue to gain weight. Two people at the same weight feel completely differently, and it all depends on where their mental attitude and image is. You can be overweight and not feel fat. Take yourself at your present weight; some days you feel fat and others you don't. Why is that? It's a mindset. Depending on how you are feeling on any given day, your mood dictates how you eat.

Some people think that if there is a special function or it's a holiday and food is abundant, they need to wear something tight. It reminds them not to overeat. Find what works for you and do it. However, I think wearing tight clothes is the worst advice. When clothes are too tight, you *feel* fat regardless of your current weight. When you feel fat, you tend to overeat. Remember, feeling fat is derogatory, and when we start to degrade ourselves, we punish ourselves with food.

When you have a function to attend or a holiday is approaching, you should really plan what you will wear. Wear something well tailored and fashionable. Your clothing and the way it fits your body dictate how you feel, and that will continually remind you of your commitment to yourself and eating better. This inspiring feeling will keep you focused on making choices best suited for you. This means you will enjoy what you eat, while you enjoy the event.

You don't have to be at your ideal body weight to feel good, but you must feel good to get to your ideal body weight. In order to feel good, you can't feel *fat*. However, that's an inside job. Now is the time to make up your mind to never again define yourself as fat.

Look back into that imaginary mirror. What do you really see? I'm sure you see things that no one else sees in you. I bet you see things that may not even be there. Let me tell you a story. It has nothing to do with weight loss/ weight management, but everything to do with what our minds see and how they play tricks on us. It was definitely an eye opener for me.

Some years ago, I attended a workshop where the theme was how to accept our body and accentuate the positive. During this workshop, we were asked to break into pairs, and I partnered with another woman. I didn't know her nor did she know me. We were asked a series of questions, which we were to answer to our partner. One question was: "What is it about your body you cannot change and have to learn to accept?" My answer was obvious to me, and I immediately said, "This large freckle on the side of my nose." My partner looked at me and said, "What large freckle on the side of your nose?" "*How* can you not see this?" I said, pointing to the right side of my nose. She said, "Margaret, I don't see a freckle." I admitted to her that each morning I cover it with makeup to dull its appearance, but insisted that it was definitely there and took up the entire side of my nose.

Then, she pulled a mirror out of her purse, probably thinking one of us was crazy and wanting to prove it wasn't her. She said, "Show me your freckle." I took the mirror and looked at my nose. Absolutely stunned, I said, "Where did my freckle go?"

When I was a young girl, I had a freckle that was darker than the other ones and almost the size of the side of my nose. Every morning until that morning when I was in my mid-forties, I saw the freckle in the mirror and covered it with extra makeup. When did that freckle disappear? Was it that morning? Probably not! When? It could have been days, weeks, months, or even years ago. Who knows? I only knew it was no longer there. However, my mind had seen it each day, and I had continued to cover it with makeup each day. I had believed the freckle was there, so it seemed it was. It took someone else to point out to me that it was gone. I no longer needed to cover that freckle with makeup. I already had what I had always wanted: a freckle-free nose!

When you look in the mirror, you need to address what's really there, not what you perceive to be there. You may need the help of others to discern your image. Maybe you need to be honest with yourself. What three words do you think defines your body image? Whatever they are, you will make them your reality. As long as you believe those words, you will live them.

One of my clients, a woman in her sixties, had attended Overeaters Anonymous (OA) meetings in her younger years. They had taught her that she was a compulsive overeater. She was encouraged to stand, announce her name, and say, "I'm a compulsive overeater." This label stayed with her for too many years. She believed this and as long as she believed it, she lived it. This label had been doing her harm. It was time to shed "compulsive overeater." However, doing this was hard for her. Her belief was deep. We discussed alternate labels that she could embrace. One day I suggested, "Why don't you consider yourself a survivor?" That changed her entire perspective. "I am a survivor," she announced over and again. That became her new three words: "I'm a survivor."

Shortly after this, a twenty-nine-year-old client whom I was seeing weekly told me that she also attended OA meetings on a regular basis. She announced to me: "I'm a compulsive overeater." I told her the story of the other woman and, hoping to shorten her learning curve, suggested she should not label herself as such. I suggested that she go to her next OA meeting, state her name, and then say, "I am eating healthily today." The first time she said it, people looked at her oddly, but after a few meetings others began saying the same thing. Her new three words became: "I eat well."

One client is a surgical nurse, and at one of our meetings she confided to me the difficult time she had making choices regarding her eating. For years, she berated herself and abused her body, believing she was not capable of having a positive attitude and healthy mindset. I asked her how often in her professional life she had had to make a split-second decision. "Always," was her reply. I continued, "Well, if you can make a split-second decision on someone else's behalf, what's stopping you from practicing that same type of decision-making for your own benefit?" That was the light-bulb moment for her. Her face lit up as her mind raced. I let the thought sink in and said, "You said you are capable of making split-second decisions; you've been doing it for years. Now you need to benefit from that skill that you already own." Her new words to describe herself became "capable of split-second decisions." (Okay, in this case, it was four words.)

In my childhood, my brothers called me: "Margaret, Margaret, the big fat target!" Today I can laugh, but for many years I cried about it. What's interesting is, during all the years I cried about it, I also believed it. Hence, the crying, and, as long as I believed it, I lived it.

That's how I had defined my body image and my self-image through my childhood, adolescence, and most of my twenties: "Margaret, Margaret, the big fat target!" Maybe the words changed a bit in my head, but that was my image. No wonder I spent my twenties yo-yo dieting! I still believed I was: "Margaret, Margaret, the big fat target!" That is who I thought I was and my destiny was, so it makes sense that yo-yo dieting was my pattern.

Sometimes, I wonder why I allowed my brothers' stupid little childhood poem to shape my image. I gave that poem more power than I gave myself for too many years, so much power that I shrugged off any compliment I received!

Who or what created the body image you have today? Was it all you? I don't think so. It was, in all probability, a combination of situations and/or people in your life. If your body image today is not one that allows you to move forward, it's time for a change. If you are stuck in a negative image, realize that it's you keeping you there, and it's you who can erase it! Body image and self-image is your perception. Change your perception, and you will find confidence you never knew you had.

Once I had decided to create a new perception, I was able to redefine my body image. This change was not immediate. It took a realization of what I wanted to be. I captured the essence of someone I admired, Princess Diana. She and I have the same birth date, July 1. She was married two months after me, but it was *I* who married the prince. What was it about Princess Diana that had impressed me? I came up with three words. I had found her to be eloquent, graceful, and feminine. As years passed, I realized Princess Diana probably did not perceive herself to be eloquent, graceful, and feminine, but this was my perception of her. In time, we came to learn of her sad life, the demons that tortured her, and her tragic death. Being a princess does not protect you from some things.

Eloquent, graceful, and feminine are not words that would have defined me earlier in my life. Remember, growing up, I was an only girl with four brothers, and I could be as rough and tumble as they were. I was like a bull in a china shop. If I wanted to become eloquent, graceful, and feminine, I had to change my attitudes and my ways. Now, do these three words have anything at all to do with my body weight? No! Yet, they have everything to do with it. How could I be "Margaret, Margaret, the big fat target!" and eloquent, graceful, and feminine at the same time? I couldn't. I had to change my perception. How could "Margaret, Margaret, the big fat target!" stand in front of a room of people who had come to gain insights and direction in their lives? She couldn't. But, today's Margaret can. I believe eloquent, graceful, and feminine is a powerful self-image. It's also an attitude.

Our attitudes control our lives. Attitudes are the secret power working twenty-four hours a day for good or bad. Your attitude is 100 percent of everything you do. Your attitude guides you. Do you need an attitude adjustment? I did.

At the time of my metamorphosis, I was heavier than I had ever been, and getting still heavier. At that time, I wore a red bathrobe all day and never put on makeup or jewelry. I didn't shower or do my hair until later in the afternoon. I would just throw anything comfortable on for the rest of the day. I was a stay-at-home mom with two little ones. Wasn't that a wonderful excuse not to take care of myself? Once my body image/self-image changed, everything changed. I began to live as if I were eloquent, graceful, and feminine. It did not mean I had to wear the gowns and tiaras that Princess Diana had worn. (Wouldn't that have been fun?) However, it took practice.

Changing my image also meant a change of attitude. Once I adopted that attitude, my body image changed to a body I wanted to nurture and take good care of, and then my eating changed.

One of the first things I changed was how and when I dressed. I began to shower, do my hair, and put on makeup and jewelry first thing every morning. Sometimes, I did all this before the kids were awake! I dressed for me. I stopped wearing sneakers and wore shoes. Eventually, I even threw out that red bathrobe!

Next, I learned to eat right and have healthier foods in the house. Finally, I exercised daily. I became more involved in outside activities and made new friends. Now I wasn't dressing only for me, I was dressing because I was going somewhere. It's funny that my children never noticed the change, but others did, and so did I.

You never know where life will take you. Eventually, helping others to realize their personal best became my passion and my life's work. Could "Margaret, Margaret, the big fat target!" have ever accomplished this? That's doubtful! Does everyone who knows me or meets me think I am eloquent, graceful, and feminine? I hope so, but it doesn't matter. It only matters to me what *I think!*

The way you feel about yourself can knock you down so low that you believe it's what you deserve and where you belong. On the other hand, the way you feel about yourself can build self-confidence and a positive body image, which can propel you to a higher level of self-esteem. To achieve the latter, dress well and treat your body well. What you feel on the inside, you show on the outside. Unlock your potential and create healthy, winning attitudes. Be who you truly want to be. Your personal mission is a statement of who you will be and what you will do to make it your reality.

Listen to unsolicited comments from others. There is a wealth of information in them. Keep a log of unsolicited comments. Every time you hear a comment or compliment, write it down. A picture begins to form. It may be a picture you want to change or a picture you want to embrace and own. It may even be a picture of which you are not aware. You'll find some people make comments from their own insecurities or jealousy. Consider the source of the comments before you give them power.

Wear special-occasion clothes everyday, and you will feel special. When you make yourself *feel* special, you *are* special, and you treat yourself so. It only matters what *you* think! *You* decide what goes in your body and on it. The unsolicited comments and compliments may give you a general picture, but you control the paintbrush in your picture. You can continue to create new images throughout each cycle of your life!

As your body image changes and you begin living a new image and losing weight, it is vital to lose the old clothes and old images that keep giving you old messages. They are no longer needed. Realize the importance of feeling magnificent throughout the entire weight-loss process. Wearing clothes that are too big and hang too loose on your body does not and will not encourage feelings of self-worth.

If you have a lot of weight to lose and do not want to invest in new clothes every time you drop a size, shop at thrift shops until you are in the size you desire. Wearing clothes that fit your body will give you a whole new perspective, build your self-confidence, and encourage you to continue your weight-loss process. When the time is right, invest in the clothes and accessories you have always wanted from the stores in which you always dreamed of shopping!

The key to keeping your new image is to continually focus on things that allow that image to flourish. This is amazingly simple when you believe your new image.

A client in her forties had a sister who was always called "the skinny sister," making my client—in her mind—the opposite. This client's self-image has always been: "The heavy sister." I had never met "the skinny sister" or even heard about her until the day my client became: "The skinny sister." She stepped on the scale and shrieked, "Today I weigh less than my sister!"

My client shared her feelings about all the years she spent as "the heavy sister." (Although she used the *fat* word, I've substituted that for heavy). What she admitted to me was magical. She said, "After spending years wishing my sister would *gain* weight, I was finally able to take control and work on myself to *lose* weight." To help her create a new body image and self-image, we had to take the sister out of the equation. A confident person has no need to compare themselves to others. My client had to create an entirely new image of herself, independent from her sister. She had to find an image that fit her life now. Her new three words to describe herself were: "Vibrant, active individual." She continues to live that image.

Look in the mirror again. What are your new three words? Is there someone you would like to emulate? Be aware you can never be that person nor should you want to be. Besides, in spite of how well you think you know a person, who that person really is, how they think, and how they act are unknown to you When you compare yourself to another, you only see the tip of their iceberg and you rob yourself of your own joy.

I admit to still reading books about Princess Diana and looking with admiration at the pictures. She was a classic beauty. Nonetheless, I'll take my life over Princess Diana's any day.

At the start of my seminars, I sometimes ask attendees to consider three words that define their self-image. Before the end of the presentation, I ask them for a new three words, which will define what you really want to achieve. One man, who was unwilling to share his first three, shared the new three words he had chosen to describe his new body image: "I really thought about this and what I want to see in that mirror is 'fit, energetic, and peaceful.'" He went on to say, "These words are a total turn-around from an hour ago." However, he voiced concern that "fit" and "energetic" do not seem to go with "peaceful." "Oh, quite the contrary," I said. "There is an enormous amount of peace when you are fit and energetic!" I believe he left that evening with a new self-image. I wish that for you, too!

While having lunch at a convention where I was scheduled to speak, I sat with a very nice, overweight gentleman. After we introduced ourselves to each other, he realized I was one of the speakers presenting a breakout session at his company's invitation. My session was entitled: "Wellness in the Workplace is Contagious." He asked me to give him three pieces of advice about his body weight. I looked him straight in the eye, and said, *"Knowledge, patience, and practice,* and without patience you have no practice." He was surprised at my answer. He said that he had thought I would say something like eat vegetables or drink water. He appreciated my answer and admitted that he had very little patience, giving him no practice, and now he realizes what needs to change.

Pick your new three words and make them concrete. Decide the steps you'll take to create your reality. Commit to them. Allow nothing to sway you. Your image is your perception. You are the creator of your image, regardless of your current body weight. When you have a positive body image or self-image, you will care for yourself in a way you never imagined possible!

Points to Remember

» Fat is a derogatory state of feeling.

» Look into a mirror and only address what's really there, not what you perceive to be there.

» Your body-image/self-image is your perception; you can change your perception, today.

» Wear special-occasion clothes everyday, and you will always feel special.

What's in It for You?

Replace "I can't" with "How can I?"
—Margaret Marshall

What you think, what you do, and how you feel affects others; and how others think, what they do, and how they feel affects you. Have you ever analyzed what each one of your relationships represents to you?

Let me start with a story about a man named Robert, who is in his seventies. I met Robert at a two-night seminar I was conducting. The room was filled with men and women—some of them were couples—but Robert was the only man who came by himself. It was obvious he was at a healthy weight. While everyone else was dressed casually, he was dressed impeccably in a sport coat, slacks, dress shirt, and tie.

The first evening, Robert told me he needed to sit up front because he was hard of hearing. I watched him as the seminar unfolded. He listened intently to the weight loss- topics discussed. When someone asked a question, he turned to him or her to make sure he could hear exactly what was said. Finally Robert asked a question: "How do you change the person you are living with?" Until then, all of the group's questions had been about themselves. However, it was apparent that Robert was at this seminar to change someone he loved.

We discussed that you can't change anyone else. No one changes unless they are willing to change. This was not the answer he had wanted. He had hoped to take home words of wisdom to change the person with whom he lives. He seemed deflated.

After the seminar, Robert shook my hand and spoke with me privately. He told me that he eats right, exercises, and generally takes good care of himself. However, his wife is overweight. He said he knows exactly what she should do to lose weight, and he can't understand why she won't do exactly what he advises. He explained that he is a retired engineer and everything to him is black and white. "I understand," I said, "but weight loss is never black and white. There is an awful lot of grey." I asked him to return the following evening for the conclusion of the seminar. He said, "Tomorrow night you are talking about relationships?" Then, he waved his hand at my face and continued, "I have no relationships; it's just me and my wife. We have no one else." "It was a pleasure to meet you," I said, and "I do hope to see you tomorrow evening." We parted ways.

The next evening I arrived early to set up the room, and I was surprised to see Robert, the first person to arrive. He claimed his seat up front. Once again, he was dressed professionally. I welcomed him and said, "I'm so glad to see you again."

As planned, the final topic discussed that evening was relationships. Robert sat and listened intently to the two-hour seminar and never spoke or asked a question. At the completion, he approached me to speak privately again. He thanked me for the valuable information and said, "I now recognize people really struggle with this. It is not easy for most of them, and I never realized that before." Now that he understood weight loss was not just a black and white issue, he would be more understanding of his wife. Between us, we agreed that all diets look good on paper; the challenge is the implementation.

Just the night before, Robert had waved his hand in my face and claimed that he had no relationships. The wave of his hand signaled that his coming the next evening would be worthless and a waste of his time! In reality, by attending, he improved the most important relationship in his entire life because *he* changed. *He* was now open to understanding the trials his wife encountered daily with her eating and body weight.

How often do our loved ones tell us what they think we need to do about our eating? My guess is that one of the reasons Robert's wife is overweight is *because* of his insistence that she do what *he* thinks is right. Most likely, she became resistant, defiant, and belligerent, which led to constant overeating. (I see this often in families, especially in adolescents.) If you have someone like Robert in your life, are they a supporter or a saboteur? They may believe they have your best interest in mind. But in reality, are they supporting you or are they are actually sabotaging you?

Nobody wants to be told what to do. When you warn a young child, "Do not touch!" something, they immediately try to figure out how to touch it without getting caught. When it comes to food, you always get caught; it shows on your body. If you feel resistant, defiant, and belligerent, you will continue to gain weight.

Evaluate all of your relationships. How does food and eating play a part in these relationships? One client, a young woman who has never been married, said to me one evening, "When I get married, I want to marry someone who doesn't care if I put on weight over the years." I told her, "I get that and that would be admirable. I know if I had spent my life gaining weight, Chris would still love me." I'm very confident in that statement. On the other hand, I explained: "Our lives would have been so different. We would not have been able to enjoy all that we have done together. Our family dynamics would not have been the same. We probably would have had to deal with illnesses and injuries throughout the years. My kids would have had a completely different childhood." The look of acceptance on her face indicated to me that she had finally realized she needed to take care of herself not only for herself, but also for the benefit of those around her!

On the first night I was working with her, still another client was depressed and feeling out of control with her life and her eating. I asked her that first evening to write down how she was feeling. Now, every once in a while, I read to her what she had written back then. She remembers feeling that way and cringes with the memory.

"I feel horrible," she wrote. "I find it very hard to get around or even do normal everyday things. My knee really hurts badly. I don't want to go anywhere. I feel like I am missing out on so much, and it gets very depressing. I feel like I'm not living my life, just existing. I just want to feel like I have some energy so I won't be so lazy."

Another client, who was in her fifties, said she realized that throughout her life she would eat too much food just because she liked it, she was bored, or whatever. It affected her family and their life together. She believes that she deprived her family of quality time and cherished memories because of her eating and weight. She now realizes that when she takes care of herself, everyone benefits!

One client, a woman in her thirties, claims she has "clarity of thought" when she avoids overeating sweets. Each day, she keeps a journal of her thoughts and feelings. Working together, we pay particular attention to when sweets begin to creep back into her week. Through this practice, she has discovered that the common denominator of much of her sweets eating is that it occurs when she visits her parents' home, where she was raised. On each visit, she would return to eating the sweets her parents always had available when she was growing up and continue to have on hand today.

Although already aware of this phenomenon, she had ignored it. Through journaling, she was able to understand it, address it, and reconstruct her visits to her family's home.

What about the parent/child relationship? A parent can support wellness efforts or sabotage the efforts of family members. One client, a busy attorney with a young son, said she likes the ease of fast-food restaurants. Besides, she said, she had not felt the need to be as thin as a super-model, so she had believed she could eat fast food regularly. However, now, she is concerned because fast food is the only dinner her five-year-old son will eat! In addition, she has been steadily gaining weight due to this lifestyle choice. Finally, she realized that she *is* a super-model... to her son! Children model the behavior of their parents and only know what is familiar to them. My client was modeling poor food choices and an overweight existence.

According to a woman at my seminar, she had been so busy, "keeping up with the Jones," that she had neglected the health of herself and her family for years. Now, she realizes that although she had attained materialistic trappings, she and her children had become overweight and unhealthy.

Another client lamented that whenever she goes grocery shopping, her son continually asks her to buy candy. To quiet him, she buys it. Then, once they are home, she eats it before her son does, because "candy is not good for him." Do you think she is really making the purchase for her son?

Who is sabotaging these families? Are these mothers too *busy* or too *lazy?* Regardless, both busy and lazy produce the same results; their families are overweight and unhealthy. Today, childhood obesity is rampant, and children as young as six have been diagnosed with high cholesterol. Again, children model the positive or negative behavior of their parents. We need to be super-models to them, because they will model us either way!

Think about you, take care of you, and acknowledge your eating patterns. It's amazing how your behavior can affect the behavior of others around you. It may take years for them to change, but it can and does happen.

When I started seriously losing weight, I was involved in a playgroup. My playgroup consisted of five young mothers with small children. We met once a week and took turns hosting. We had lunch together while our children played. Our conversations were enthralling, and we covered every topic imaginable. Each week, I looked forward to the playgroup because not only did the kids have fun playing together, but also the camaraderie and friendship of these women were priceless to me!

Unfortunately, I began to realize that the playgroup was sabotaging my weight-loss efforts. Now, each week, I left feeling sad and angry. This had nothing to do with the other women, although it would have been easy to blame them. It was my fault. Some of our weekly conversations were about weight loss and how unhappy some of us were at our current weight. Early on, I realized I was the only one seriously working at changing my weight.

During our weekly gatherings, we enjoyed gourmet lunches. We always tried to out-do previous lunches with new recipes we found, and we succeeded. The food was delicious and abundant at these playgroups and desserts were even more so! The four women who hadn't cooked something that week brought desserts. So, every week, we had a new tantalizing lunch and four-times-too-much dessert.

Each week, I promised myself that I would control myself and *not* eat too much. (Notice the word, *not*). However, I gave in to the temptation each time. I would return home feeling sad and often spent the rest of the day—sometimes the next few days—overeating. It's the body, mind, and mouth connection. Every fifth week, when I hosted playgroup at my house, the challenge was even greater. Then, I had *four leftover desserts!* I finally realized giving up playgroup was not an option. Finding a new way of handling it was.

I explained to my playgroup friends how much I looked forward to our luncheons and how exciting it was trying all these different recipes. I let them know how important our conversations were and how much they meant to me. I also knew my friends enjoyed these luncheons as much as I did. So, I just asked that we do things a little differently.

I suggested that whoever hosts the luncheon also should be in charge of dessert. This suggestion was well received. It accomplished two things. The focus was now on the luncheon and not on all the desserts. In one week, we went from four desserts to one. I decided that on playgroup days my lunch would be my main meal. Later that evening, I would eat something smaller. I also knew I could enjoy a small piece of dessert that afternoon and not feel bad about it—clarity of thought! I had taken control.

When I asked my friends for this change, I never once mentioned the struggles I had had with my weight. We implemented our new luncheon menu and enjoyed playgroup for a few more years. When the kids reached school age, playgroup ended, but I had learned a valuable lesson. We all have the ability to create scenarios that work for us. Today, I look back at playgroup with fond memories and encourage young mothers to establish strong relationships with other young mothers.

In order for these scenarios to be successful, everyone must be considered. I never went to my playgroup moms and asked that they eliminate food because I had found it too hard to control. They would lose *me* before the food! Honestly, I did not want that either. I simply asked whether it might be easier if the person making lunch might also make dessert. No further explanation was needed.

If you tell someone, "I can't eat this item, I'm trying to lose weight, or I'm dieting," what you are really saying is, "Twist my arm a little harder, and I'll eat with you." It becomes a challenge to others to see how strong-willed you can be. When you eat every time someone wants you to eat or because someone puts food in front of you, you will gain your weight and their weight, too.

We show people how to treat us, we don't tell them. If you continually tell someone you're dieting, but your actions say otherwise, nobody listens.

One client couldn't understand why her grandmother kept making her favorite baked goods, "especially for her," as Grandma would say. She had told her grandmother many times she is trying to lose weight, but food is love! Many people show their love with food. Grandma was showing her granddaughter how much she loves her with food.

In our sessions, we had discussed this many times. Now, we have a strategy in place for my client to counteract Grandma's baking while still allowing her grandmother to show her love. You can't change anyone else. You can only change yourself and you never want to hurt anyone you love, especially Grandma, for showing you her love.

We came up with the plan after my client had recounted another visit to Grandma. This time, my client's sister had accompanied her. Again, Grandma baked my client's favorite biscuits. She asked her grandmother why she hadn't asked her sister to have biscuits. Grandma replied, "Oh, I know she is always watching her weight." This comment angered and astounded my client. It didn't help that her sister weighed less than she did. My client said she felt as if her grandmother had said to her, "Your sister is thin and you are already fat (her word), so what difference does it make?" Of course, Grandma had said nothing of the kind!

I suggested we look at this scenario from a different angle. I asked her if her sister would have accepted Grandma's offer of a biscuit. She didn't know, so she asked her sister. Her sister's reply was, "No way! They are too heavy." My client needed to realize that she talked the talk, but didn't walk the walk. Grandma knows which granddaughter eats the baked goods and which one does not. She realized that her grandmother's actions did not say, "You're already fat," they said, "You always show me you like this, and I like making you happy." We agreed that nobody likes to be told no, and Grandma knew that my client's sister would turn down her offer of a biscuit.

This client finally realized her words needed to match her actions. You can tell people what you want to achieve, but they only listen when you show them. Years ago, I realized that it was good to say, "No thank you—not now, maybe later," or "No thank you—I'm good," which were easier for the other person to accept. They stopped pushing food. That statement now rolls off my tongue. I've had a lot of practice. These statements are for my wellness, and the eating patterns I developed and desire.

I've learned to nurture the relationships that are beneficial to my well-being. Sometimes, I have to reevaluate a relationship, which might change the importance of that relationship. There are also times I have to step away from a relationship. When you realize that taking care of yourself is serious business, you may find there are some relationships you no longer want to continue. If that's the case, maybe the relationship is more toxic than you thought, and it is probably in your best interest to end it. At times, you'll also find that some people are just hurting, and they soothe their hurt by hurting you. Keep your distance from them until it passes.

If you feel you are being sabotaged by a relationship, become aware of the part you play in it. Your part is larger than anyone else's could ever be. Once you understand your part, you can refocus, redefine, and then re-engage in your relationship. It's your actions that are most important.

People will come in and out of your life. Some are supportive to your weight-loss and wellness efforts. They understand and instinctively know what your needs are. It could be because they have been there. Maybe they just want the best for you. Know your part in that relationship as well. Chances are, you instinctively know what their needs are and treat these people appropriately. Look to them for support.

Some will never support your wellness efforts. They don't understand, don't care, or don't have the time. You may never know why. Sometimes they are unhappy or overwhelmed themselves and have nothing to give anyone else. You need to accept them for who they are and look to others for support. You are the most important component in any of your relationships.

Think about what attracts you to others. Make a list of attributes you admire in others. You might find that you have similar attributes. What you admire in others is what they admire in you.

I find I'm attracted to people with big smiles. There is something warm and welcoming in a smile. Many have told me that I have a bright, wide smile. Most often, I don't know I'm smiling. After I hear this comment, I sure feel that smile.

Points to Remember

- The most important relationship is the one you have with yourself.
- Your wellness is serious business.
- It is your actions that are most important.
- If you eat every time someone else wants you to, you will gain his or her weight, too.

Your Inner Dialogue

"You talkin' to me?"
—Robert DeNiro, Taxi Driver, 1976

You are the result today of all of your past experiences. Everything in your life has led you to this moment. Every diet you have ever tried led you to the weight you are today. Every thought you have ever had in the past controls your thought process now. You have worked hard to get where you are, whether you like where you are or not.

You have either watched people in your life and said to yourself, "I want to be just like him/her, or I don't want to be anything like them." They taught you how to think, feel, or act; or showed you how not to think, feel, or act. Who do you think you are most like? Is that who you want to be?

My father was heavy, and when I was a child he would say to me, "Margaret, you and I will fight the battle of the bulge together." While I understand that he was trying to inspire me to watch my weight, his words contributed to a belief system that I will always be heavy.

One day, I attended a bridal shower with my mom and my then-toddler daughter, Megan. My mom looked great and received many compliments. Everyone told Megan how cute she was. On the other hand, not one kind comment or compliment came my way. The silence was deafening. The "no comment" screamed: "Margaret, you're frumpy, and maybe you should do something about that."

Is that what others really thought? Probably not! In any case, that's what I thought. I knew my definition of myself had to change. I did not want to be heavy my entire life. I had often been told that I was "big-boned." That was another one of my belief systems, big-boned or large. So what! Even if I did have "big bones," I didn't need excess body fat on my "big bones."

When I changed the message to myself, I changed my weight. Every diet I had been on gave me internal messages that said, "Weight loss is temporary." In reality, when you take care of yourself in every area, at all times, and when you respect and love yourself, weight loss can and will be permanent.

Self-love is never selfish. You can't love anyone else without loving yourself, and you can't offer others a deeper love than the love you have for yourself.

Does this mean I am never challenged with food situations, or that my weight is always exactly the same? Never! It means I'm up for the challenge, and it's worth it!

Do you realize you have about 50,000 thoughts a day? Are the vast majority of them negative thoughts?

Examples:

- I'm not as good as...
- I'm not as smart as...
- I'll never be able to...
- I'm not as pretty or handsome as, or built like...
- I'll never lose this weight.

» I'll always be this weight.

» Etc., etc., etc.!

With all that negativity going on in our heads, how do we get anything accomplished? For one day, note the thoughts you have during that day. Keep a pen and pad handy. Write them all down. Be honest with yourself. Write every thought, not just the ones you want to admit. As you read your list of thoughts, you might think, I need to get out of here! That's exactly what you are doing, getting outside of your thoughts and looking in from the outside. Until you become aware of them, you can't change your thoughts. See them and hear them.

How many of your thoughts are negative? Would you say those things to anyone else? If you talked like that to a friend, you would be friendless and lead a lonely life. Try telling a friend that she is not as pretty or as smart as someone else. See how long they remain your friend. Why do *you* deserve to be spoken to like that? Say out loud, to yourself, in an indignant tone with an exaggerated New York accent: *"You talkin' to me?"*(As Robert De Niro, portraying, Travis Bickle, in Taxi Driver, said.) Then, *stop* talking to yourself that way!

Have you ever had a day when you feel sad or bad and don't know why? Could it be your thoughts? They are constantly there, constantly dictating how you feel, and influencing how you eat. Your thoughts guide you all day, without your permission. Thoughts lead to feelings, and feelings can dictate eating.

Are you stressed? Stress proves you are alive. Do you believe situations in your life causes you stress? Stress is how we internally think and feel about each situation.

Stress is always a feeling, not a situation. Does stress lead you to eat?

Two people can have the same situation; one is stressed, while the other is not. If you are aware of how you think and feel, you can react in a proactive way. If you are stressed, you are allowing thoughts and feelings to build up inside you with no ending.

You can change your stress by becoming aware of it and changing your thoughts. You feel stress, so you think sweets. You can stop that cycle today.

Become aware of your thoughts and you can control your feelings. It sounds simple, but it's not! You need to continually practice this, but it is worth the effort! It's the body, mind, and mouth connection.

When I was at that bridal shower with my mom and daughter, not one person said I looked frumpy. That is only what I thought they were thinking. Because I thought it, I began to feel and act frumpy. I'm the one who made it a reality. I hear over and over from clients how they fear what others think of them. Some examples are:

» I can't take a walk in my neighborhood. People will think: "All this walking and you still have a big butt!"

» I don't accept invitations for dinner because people will think I'll break their chairs.

» I can't go to the mall. When I do, people stare at me and wonder why I'm shopping in the same stores they do.

» When my daughter gets candy in a party bag, people think I will eat it before she does.

» Someone in a business meeting looked at me and thought I was too *fat* (their word).

» I can't order diet coke in a restaurant because people think it's funny that someone my size drinks a diet drink.

» I can't have lunch by myself because people will look at me and think I have no friends.

Again, that word, *fat,* keeps rearing its ugly head. I could give more examples, but I'm sure you have your own. Why do you believe you are an expert on another person's thoughts? You have no idea what anyone else thinks unless they tell you. Besides, who cares what others think? I know *you* care, but should you? Isn't being the best you can be enough? You can't please everyone all of the time, but you can always please yourself. Others' opinion of you is none of your business.

I believe that others have their own agenda and their own personal problems or issues. Do you really believe they want to be bogged down with yours? When you avoid something you want because of what others think, you are really avoiding it because of what you think.

To use the last example, the real fear in this individual is that she thinks she has no friends. Her self-talk might be: "Because of my weight, I am not worthy of friends and everyone knows that." To have a friend, you must be a friend, and create a friendly atmosphere for others. How sad that anyone would ever let his or her weight get in the way of a solid friendship! When invited to a party or reunion, many people stay home because of how they perceive others will think of them. These people miss out on life.

Years ago, when I went to my twentieth high school reunion, I thought, "Wow, the guys got older-looking, but the gals looked great." Then I realized that the only gals attending were those who wanted to be seen. The rest of them stayed home. I wondered how many occasions I missed because of how I felt about myself.

When you strive to please everyone, often the one person you are not pleasing is yourself. If you stay home because you fear what others think, say to yourself: "So what!" Then, go anyway. You are missing out on life, your life. Work through the feelings, and have a good time. Remember your self-love, and keep in mind that no one is perfect. Unfortunately, everyone has issues. Some people's issues are just more visible than others.

Work on your own thoughts and feelings. I realize others can influence you, but it is always *your* thoughts, feelings, and actions that control you and that you can control. Improve your relationship with yourself. You'll find in doing so, you'll improve your relationships with others.

There was a time when walking into a roomful of strangers intimidated me, so I avoided the situation at all costs. This stress was caused by my own thoughts and insecurities. One day, someone gave me great advice. Now, I'm asking you to take my advice and practice the following.

Before you walk into a party, dinner, restaurant, business meeting, reunion, or even a bridal shower, say to yourself: "These people are so lucky to have me here!" Then walk in, believing it. It works! Whenever I go to places I've never been before, I practice this, and then I can talk with people I've never met with an air of confidence.

Your overall success is in direct relationship to your strengths and weaknesses, and your strengths will only take you as far as your weaknesses allow. What are your weaknesses? If you think about it, I'm sure you can make a long list. Study that list and examine each of your weaknesses. Then, delete the ones you know, in your heart, are not true.

How do I know you'll list weaknesses that are not factual? We are always too tough on ourselves. Referring to that list again, note each of the weaknesses that are left, and think about how you exhibit each trait. For example, my list would say "lack of commitment." But when it comes to my clients, I know I am 100 percent committed to their success and well-being, sometimes more than they are! However, I am not always 100 percent committed to my own well-being. My list might also include "failure to follow through." Nonetheless, I can be very persistent when I'm trying to accomplish something for a family member. I'm suggesting that something you consider a weakness may be your strength in another area. Make it a strength in the area you need it. You already own it, and are not using it to its full potential.

Now ask a trusted friend or family member to make a list of all your strengths. Getting a loved one to create the list will make it more realistic, which can bring great insight. How many of the traits on your list of weaknesses are the same as their list of your strengths? How many traits did your loved one list that you have never even considered in defining yourself? You may not recognize what others see clearly.

If the two lists differ, you have a lot of work to do. If the two lists are similar, you need to realize and acknowledge you already have those traits. Enhance who you are with what you already have. It's naturally you. From here on, begin to fully use your individual traits as strengths to benefit yourself in every aspect of your life.

Points to Remember

- Others taught you how or how not to think, feel, and act.
- You can't please everyone all the time, but you can please yourself.
- When you respect and love yourself, weight loss can and will be permanent.
- Thoughts lead to feelings and feelings lead to overeating.

Eat What You Like; Learn How to Eat It

Healthy eating: eating foods that are enjoyable to you, in the quantity that is good for you.
—Margaret Marshall

"I know what to do; I just have to do it." Have you heard yourself say this time and time again? Do you really know what to do? How many different diets have you tried? Have you ever noticed that ads for the latest diets, pills, or surgeries always state "along with a balanced diet" or "results not typical"?

How many times have you tried the same commercial diet plan because of the actress touting her success, the registration is free, you'll receive a free giveaway, or there's a discount on packaged food? The odds are your dedication to that diet plan was short-lived because it was born from commercialism. How many times have you re-visited the same diet program and each time you started, you were a little heavier? Have you read the labels on the diet industry's so-called diet food? If you can't pronounce the ingredients, why are you eating them? Have you seen the list of the top ten scams in our country? Weight-loss products promising dramatic results are on that list. Common sense is the best approach to sustained weight loss and optimal health, yet it's the method least used.

You possess within you everything needed for a healthy body weight and sustained weight management. You have your brain for knowledge, reason, and self-love; your body to move; and your mouth to feed. With knowledge, you will instinctively know what works for you. Reason will help you to sort through all the hype, myths, and marketing ploys so you don't waste your time and resources. Self-love will constantly keep you aware of the importance of caring for yourself. *Knowledge* and *reason,* along with *self-love,* will guide your mouth to feed, nourish, and nurture your body to sustain your life.

Maybe you know what to do, but you just don't know how to implement your plan. I know there are always extenuating circumstances. Forget them and live as if they don't exist. They are only as powerful as you make them. If you're waiting for the perfect time or until you are ready, your may never achieve a healthy body weight. *Capture the moment, and make now the perfect time.*

In order to succeed at living a thin healthy life, you need to make the way you eat who you *are* and not what you *do.* It already is: the way you eat *is* who you are. The question is: Is that who you want to be anymore? When you implement and embrace a lifestyle of healthy eating, you will be healthier. Healthy eating does not mean eating grilled chicken and string beans. It means learning how to eat foods that you enjoy and that will also nourish your body. It means eating the quantity of food that is right for your body size, and it means getting pleasure from everything you eat. When this becomes who you are, you will have a healthier body inside and out.

You don't have to give up your favorite foods. However, if there are foods that prevent you from getting where you want to be, reevaluate what these foods mean to you. Put them in their place, and then treat them accordingly. In addition, you will need to eliminate any eating or drinking patterns that steal more energy than they create.

Do the foods you eat each day work for or against you? If they work against you, but you still love these foods, decide how you can make them special instead of a staple in your everyday diet. When you make them special, you will savor and enjoy them more.

You crave what you are most accustomed to feeding your body. If you frequently eat high-sugar content foods, fast food, or drink alcohol, these are the items you find yourself craving. When you become familiar with eating more quality foods or drinking water, your body will begin to crave these items. Clients are always astounded at this concept. When they give it time, new habits develop, and then they say, "I never thought I would be craving salads, fruits, or water!" In the past, they hadn't given it enough time. At the very first craving of sugar or whatever, they gave in, and gave up. No more!

At various times of your life, you may find that different foods hold different value. When I was a young girl, I couldn't dream of never having another Ring Ding, yet today I would never think of having one. We eat differently depending on our age. Foods that once held you spellbound may no longer have any effect. Many items that we ate in our childhood should not follow us into our adult life. If we leave childhood games and ideas behind, shouldn't we also leave the childhood food as well?

Some of what we ate and drank in our twenties does not belong in our thirties. As you leave the forties and enter the fifties, eating needs to change yet again. For instance, menopausal women find that their bodies begin to react differently to certain foods. As we enter into our sixties, seventies, and beyond, our eating and tastes will change again. Throughout the later years, a number of us may have to follow different dietary guidelines due to medical reasons.

Each cycle of life brings a different eating style. As you age, your body metabolizes food differently. You may observe that a particular food item does not taste the same as it did twenty years ago. What changed: you or the food item? Acknowledge the foods that you once thought were incredible, but no longer enjoy. Put them out of your mind, and take them out of your daily diet.

We hold onto the memory of some foods. Although we may cherish the memory, the food item may no longer have true value. When clients are asked to temporarily delete a particular food item from their daily diet because it's standing in the way of their progress, they usually realize the enjoyment of that food is attached to a memory. With this awareness, they can now let go of the desire for the item. They begin to understand that tastes, desires, and cravings change with age.

At times, do you ask yourself, "*What* can I eat?" Change your question to, "*Why* do I feel like eating?" When you change your *what* to a *why*, you get different insight, which leads to another answer and a changed direction.

A client told me she and her family had had pizza for dinner; she had planned on having two slices for dinner and did. After dinner, she began cleaning the kitchen. There was one slice of pizza left in the box. Alone in the kitchen, she ate the last slice. She should have asked herself: "Why do I want this slice of pizza?" She had enjoyed the two slices she ate with her family. These were planned and special, but, without a doubt, that third slice was eaten fast and secretly. Think how often and how much you eat secretly, and why you do that. Acknowledge what secret eating does to your weight and mindset.

I grew up with four brothers. When I was young, if there was food in the refrigerator that I might want, even if I didn't want it at that moment, I would eat it anyway. With all those brothers, I knew if I didn't eat the food then, it wouldn't be there when I did want it. I learned at a young age to eat it now, eat it fast, and eat it secretly. That pattern followed me for more years than I care to admit. As an adult, living in my own home, no one was going to take the food. However, until I became aware of my groundless fear, I still ate as if the item wouldn't be there later. When times change, change the eating patterns. Everything you do, and everything you eat, matters.

Your body is your temple, and it needs to have a strong foundation, that comes from proper care and good, healthy eating. Would you build the house of your dreams on a shaky foundation? Of course you wouldn't! It would be worthless, couldn't last, and would give you more problems than joy. In time, it would crumble and become useless. You would spend too much of your time and resources repairing it.

You need to think the same way about your body. Houses can be sold and you move on, leaving those problems to the poor soul who purchased it. However, you have only one body, and you don't want to be the poor soul inhabiting a body with a weak foundation.

Many overweight people ask: "How did I allow myself to get to this weight?" or "How did I get to this weight again?" or "I promised myself I would never let this happen." These people had a terrible foundation and have allowed their bodies to crumble over the years. As long as you are breathing, you can still change your situation. It's never too late. Living a thin, healthy life takes persistent, consistent action on your part.

In no way do I profess to be perfect. People say to me, "It's easy for you; you're at a healthy weight." I need to be clear about this: It's not easy; it takes the persistent, consistent action just mentioned. Weight comes back quickly, and you need to know exactly where it shows up on your body first. Not only should you look at the scale weekly, look at your body and the way your clothes fit. Be mindful of everything you eat. Know your strengths and weaknesses, and how to make each one work *for* you, not against you. This takes persistence and practice, not perfection.

Persistence requires a definite purpose and plan. Ignore negative and discouraging influences. Keep people that will encourage you close by. People tell me, in a disgruntled tone, that I have no idea how it feels to be 100 or more pounds overweight. Thankfully, they are correct! But I do know what it is like to manage, care for, and preserve my weight every day of my adult life. Never apologize; strive.

Some people say, "It's easier to gain weight than to lose weight." Well, how can that be? How can gaining weight be easier, with all the unhappiness, physical pain, and self-abuse that usually accompany weight gain? It is easier to take a stand and take care of yourself, even during the most difficult times of your life. In the grand picture, it's the easiest path to take.

In the technology world, things change all the time. It seems that by the time you purchase and figure out how to use the latest technology, it's obsolete. In the weight-loss world, the same is *not* true. There is nothing new! It's just packaged differently. There's the most recent diet plan that includes pills, shakes, bars, diet frozen foods or diet desserts. There's counting calories, fat grams, carbs, net carbs, or points. There's even surgery. The only thing new is you. Once you decide you want a healthy body and that you are done with fads, gimmicks, packaged foods, and programs, you'll stop believing these items give you power. Then, it becomes obvious to you that it's time to care for yourself. Change will occur. There is always a choice, and you can benefit from what you choose.

Are you resistant to the common-sense approach because it takes too long to see results or you know someone who lost weight rapidly with the latest gimmick or new kind of surgery? Numerous people who have had gastric bypass or lap-band surgery have regained a large portion of their weight. They relied on the surgery to achieve the loss for them, and never changed what needed to be changed internally, deep within them.

Always look within. My clients understand that I can only guide them; I can't lose weight for them. I can only be responsible *to* them; I can't be responsible *for* them. When they have this understanding, they are on their way to change their weight and they know it. When a client tells me, "I thought a lot about what you said," from a discussion we had, it's music to my ears. They heard some tidbit of advice that changed their thinking and their actions. Thinking will continually change your actions, and actions will always change your thinking.

Albert Einstein said, "You can't solve a problem with the same mind that created it." Who created the reality of you being overweight, regardless of how overweight you are? You did. It was your thoughts and actions!

Support and encouragement are vital. It is essential to have someone you trust to help guide you, but each individual does his or her own work, every day without fail. It's time to take responsibility for your thoughts, actions, and body. You are the only one that can control your weight.

Are you tired of thinking that this is the year you will lose weight? How many New Years have begun with this wish? How many special occasions passed for which you wanted to lose weight? Weight loss does not happen by wishing. Learn what works for you now. What worked for you years ago may have changed. You need to change with the cycles of your life.

Because of past experiences with dieting, many believe the word diet has come to mean deprivation. Deprivation will never lead to weight loss. Never! Deprivation will always lead to overeating. "Diet" is simply what you eat. For example, if you eat cereal all day, you have a "diet" of cereal. If you eat healthily, you have a "healthy diet."

Since 1987, I've worked at keeping my body at a healthy weight. If I told you I never ate cake, I would be lying. Friends and family would scream, "I've seen her eat cake." There may even be some pictures floating around. I do eat cake. It is not a staple in my diet, but sometimes it's important. I eat it when I want it, not when someone or an occasion dictates I should have it.

Nobody is overweight because they eat a piece of cake occasionally; they're overweight because they eat cake regularly.

Eating satisfaction is vital to weight loss and weight management. If you are not satisfied with what you eat, you will overeat. It is important to eat what you like, and learn how to eat it. No food should be off-limits, but there should be limits on food. There is a fine line between eating and overeating. Identify that line, keep it in perspective, and be aware as years go on, the line may move. Allow it to change with the knowledge that everything changes; nothing stays the same.

Eating is sensual. Have you ever watched someone eat food they love? That's what they do; they love it. Watch their facial expressions, the way their entire body is involved, and listen to their comments while eating. Am I describing you? Me, too! We were born to eat, and chewing is an instinct. Take either one away, and we make up for it at a later time. When that time comes, we usually eat out of control.

Use a new acronym for D-I-E-T…

D-Decide (How)

I- I'll

E-Eat

T-Today

*Diet should mean. **D**ecide how **I**'ll **E**at **T**oday.*

One client said that she was taught by her mom not to eat too much. It was ingrained in her to try to eat as little as possible, and many types of food were completely off-limits and considered evil. After years of living this way, was she at her ideal body weight? No!

When we began working together, I stressed the importance of eating during the day and adding snacks between meals that included a protein item. Unknown to me, this made her uncomfortable. She mistrusted my strategy. She sent me an e-mail to tell me how frustrated she felt. She believed she should not be eating as often during the day as we planned, and she was now thinking too much about food. She neglected to tell me about her eating belief system. She hadn't realized that she still owned this belief of deprivation that her mom had instilled.

As weeks went by, she tried some techniques we discussed, and began losing weight. It was then she realized the amount of food she was asked to eat was less than she was eating all along. In the past, she focused on eating very little and was not satisfied with the foods she allowed herself to eat. Her pattern was to overeat or binge when no one was watching. She was a "secret eater." This was a revelation for her. She now looks forward to eating during the day, while being mindful about what she eats. She currently eats a variety of good, healthy foods that she enjoys, while sparingly adding other foods she once believed to be evil. This new insight was vital to her. She needed to leave her childhood-ingrained beliefs behind; they were doing her harm.

Another childhood belief that follows people is: "You must clean your plate." Why? Some beliefs are not based on facts, and today they stand in our way and work against us. If you have beliefs holding you back, question their validity. Do they stand in the way of what you truly desire and deserve? Is it time to reevaluate them and change them to more productive messages and practices?

When you are truly serious about leading a thin, healthy life and not just losing weight, you'll realize it's not a race. True weight loss is a process that takes time, just as you can't start kindergarten in September and hope to graduate from high school the next June. How prepared would you be for life? Successful body-fat loss is a learning process. Without the lessons learned on your journey, you'll have almost no chance at keeping that weight off. What you learn about yourself while healthfully losing weight, you will carry through the rest of your life. You want to lose body fat and increase muscle mass regardless of the numbers on the scale, and that takes as long as it takes.

The following is an advertisement I recently received: "M.D. Will help you rapidly lose body fat, gain lean muscle mass, live healthier & slowdown the aging process." Too many promises! Be skeptical when you see or hear the word "rapidly" when it refers to weight loss. Unfortunately, too many people buy into this!

When you are not eating the correct, balanced, nutritious diet for your body size, you will slow your metabolic rate and lose muscle along with body fat. The scale will show a loss, but it's not the loss you want.

I'm sure you've heard friends brag how quickly they are losing weight and you wonder, what's wrong with me? But if they are not eating correctly, or they cut back too much on food, they will lose muscle mass. It will show as a weight loss on the scale. Eventually they put the weight on again, adding body fat. Because they have lost muscle mass and increased body fat, their metabolic rate slows down once again. In reality, they are setting themselves up to gain weight year after year. Like a gambler, you only hear from them when they win money, you never hear how much they lost before they finally won. The person that lost weight quickly never broaches the topic publicly after he or she has gained the weight back.

Requests come from marketing companies asking me to sell their dramatic weight-loss products to my clients. Before Thanksgiving, I received this: "Commit to sharing in the 9-day program starting next Monday, right after Thanksgiving weekend. This is the perfect way to undo any turkey/stuffing/leftovers overdosing and to shed some weight before the inevitable food cornucopia that is the Christmas Season." The company was promoting a colon cleanse, but to me, the advertisement says: "Come share in my eating disorder with me." See these advertisements for what they are. Stop believing the hype and lies.

Eating well is the way to achieve a healthy body. The scale never tells the entire story. It weighs all of you, not just your body fat. This can be a particularly frustrating part of the weight-loss process. It's like reading a book and skipping every third chapter. You just don't get the whole story with the scale alone. Numbers on the scale will increase if you have just flown, are retaining water, experiencing a lack of sleep, or are stressed or constipated. Why do we allow these small temporary gains to derail our efforts and bring about negative thoughts that lead to defeated attitudes and emotions, which produce permanent weight gain? "*When you eat what you feel, you'll feel what you eat.*"

Concentrate on your actions and the number on the scale will take care of itself. When you only concentrate on the scale, you set yourself up for a lifetime of yo-yo dieting, with your weight going constantly up and down on the scale. You never move forward to achieve your ultimate goals. You need to be dedicated to the actions that allow the numbers to decrease on the scale long-term versus letting your level of dedication and motivation be dictated by any slight—probably temporary—decrease of the numbers on the scale.

Begin empowering yourself to a thin, healthy life. Empowerment is a powerful feeling. When you are empowered, there is never a need to compare yourself with anyone else.

If you have food in your house you find challenging, get it out of the house. At one time, Chris would stop on his way home from work on occasion and buy a dozen donuts. Why? TV commercials encourage you to buy a dozen donuts from this chain of donut stores. When he walked into this particular shop, he automatically thought "a dozen donuts." Marketing at its best! He would eat two that evening, and Megan and Michael would each eat one. The next day, I was left alone with eight donuts to tempt me or just eat. When it became too challenging for me, I would throw eight donuts out.

Depending on my thoughts and feelings that day, eight donuts might not be in the house at the end of the day. There were two options, get rid of them or eat them. Throwing them out was more important to me. This had nothing to with willpower, and everything to do with empowering myself to have a feel-good day.

Often clients say they cannot throw food out. I understand and respect that. Why then, do they have no problem throwing out the fresh fruits and vegetables that were purchased with good intentions, but were never eaten because there were too many sweets to tempt them in their home? Either way, excess or leftover food will go to waste. It can go to waste or to *your waist!*

Have you ever bought a real Christmas tree for Christmas? Do you keep it after the holidays so it doesn't go to waste? No! You got your money's worth using it for your Christmas decorations, and once the holiday is over, so is its usefulness. Think the same way about leftover birthday cakes and such; once the occasion is over, the leftovers have outlived their usefulness. You have already gotten your money's worth.

Everything you eat, think, and feel will show in your body weight. Each item you eat carries either a benefit or consequence. There will always be a result. Ask yourself: "If I eat this, what is the consequence to me and my health in the years to come, or will this food benefit me in my quest for a thin, healthy life?" Equipped with that answer and insight, you can then choose wisely.

When you think, it's just one day, it doesn't matter, and who cares, you continue to overeat everyday for years. Know that it does matter, and that you *should care*. There are 365 days a year to make excuses or 365 opportunities a year to take control.

It is unfair and unjust, but society is not kind to overweight individuals. Overeating is an addiction that you wear on the outside. It can and will be your demise if the addiction is allowed to control your actions throughout the years of your life. Overweight people are passed over for job opportunities or advancement to the next level in their chosen professions. Sometimes, even friendship and love relationships suffer. Overeating and continued poor eating choices throughout the cycles of your life are the route to many diseases that could have been easily avoided. Will society change its attitude? Perhaps not, but the overweight individual can change his or her plight in life by changing eating patterns. Eating can, and most likely will, determine your level of success. Begin using the 365 days each year as opportunities to increase your mobility. Eat for your health and create the change you want on a professional level. It can be done.

Points to Remember

» Everything you eat, think, and feel will show on your body.

» Know the difference between eating and overeating.

» Reevaluate what specific food items represent to you.

» Concentrate on your actions, not the scale.

And...Action!

"Exercise and application produce order in our affairs, health of body, cheerfulness of mind, and these make us precious to our friends."
—*Thomas Jefferson*

While it's true that when you eat well and eat balanced you can lose weight without exercise; conversely, you can exercise daily while not paying close attention to what you eat and never lose weight.

The real payoff comes when you put the two together. Consider exercise and good nutrition a "Dynamic Duo." In the sixties and seventies, I grew up with four brothers and one television set for the entire family. We were each allowed to pick one show to watch in the evening before bedtime. Of course, when it was time for "Batman and Robin," I was always outvoted, so we watched every episode of the original Dynamic Duo as a family. No matter what challenges the Dynamic Duo faced or what villains they fought, they always won, and the victim of the week was always freed!

The same concept is true with eating right consistently and exercising regularly. If you commit to making this your lifestyle, you'll find you will win and be free to lead a thin, healthy life. You may also find that regular exercise allows you more freedom with food choices. Consider eating healthily and performing regular daily exercise your Dynamic Duo.

During your weight-loss process, you may discover that just eating healthily is not enough to sustain long-term weight management. In order to lead a thin, healthy life, exercise is required. Your exercise should be enjoyable, beneficial, and a good fit for your lifestyle. People who have accomplished sustained weight loss throughout the years have exercised regularly.

If eating right and exercising regularly is truly the Dynamic Duo, doesn't this sound too good to be true? It sounds so easy anyone can do it. Can you? If you're not, what's stopping you? For long-term, sustained weight loss you must engage in some kind of exercise.

In presenting one of my seminars titled, "Triumph with 5 Healthy Habits," I begin the presentation stating that drinking water and exercise are *not* one of the healthy habits that we will explore and discuss. This comment confuses the audience, and after quizzical stares, comments, and further explanation, the audience realizes that if they want to live thin and be healthy, drinking water and exercising is not up for negotiation. Both are vital to good health and should be what you do, *not* what you'll think about doing.

We are all natural exercisers. When you were only a few months old, you would lie on your back and kick your feet; later in life, that is called leg lifts. Those leg lifts made you stronger and you began to crawl. Don't we marvel today at a baby who has just learned to crawl! Crawling made your arms and legs stronger. Then, you were able to pull your body up and stand holding onto a table, a form of pull-ups. What came next? Walking! Once you started to walk, there was no stopping you, and you ran!

In my childhood, we played outside. We had no video games, Facebook, or cell phones. When I wanted to play with a friend, I walked to their house and called for them by ringing their doorbell. There was no text messaging. We played hopscotch, jump rope, running bases, and stickball. We went to the park and played on monkey bars, swings, and slides. We did cartwheels, backbends, and handstands. We had races and we walked along on sidewalks attempting to "never step on a crack or you break you mother's back." There were "Red Light, Green Light: One Two Three," "Simon Says," and "Mother, May I?" In the winter we went sledding, ice-skating, and had snowball fights. This was exercise for the childhood stage of my life!

Since I lived in suburbia, after I became old enough to drive, there was no more exercise. Excuses began, and exercise stopped.

Years later, after having my two children, my motto became: "If Dairy Barn doesn't sell it, then I don't buy it." Dairy Barn is a drive-through convenience store. How convenient to purchase bread, milk, and other staples right from your car! It was much easier than enduring the hassle of putting the kids in and out of the car and walking through the grocery store with them. Then, I would return home and press a button that opened the garage door in order save a few steps and conserve energy. Yet, I always felt tired. What I didn't realize was that this wasn't saving energy. Inactivity never breeds energy. Have you ever sat on the couch for a while until you had enough energy to do your next task? What happened? Was the task accomplished? Put simply, inactivity leads to more inactivity, while activity leads to more activity. So how do you create energy in your life? Move. Start small; but start immediately!

During the process of my own weight loss, the importance of moving more became more apparent. What sports did I enjoy when I was younger? Some of those games were now unrealistic for me. One day, I mentioned to my kids that I use to do cartwheels across the backyard. They laughed and didn't believe it! So… I threw my feet into the air supported by my arms, shrieked in pain, and prayed as I hit the ground that no bones would break. Then, I realized there were no more cartwheels in my future. So, cartwheels and any other gymnastics were out. I began walking. I only walked around the block at first; this was more exercise than I had had in years.

In those days, people didn't walk everyday as they do now. It embarrassed me to be different than the norm, and God forbid someone should see me. "So what if someone sees me," I convinced myself. Soon, walking became part of my day and part of my life in all kinds of weather. This was more than twenty-five years ago.

I always walk the same route for a few reasons, safety being the most important one. When the breeze softly blows, it's like being kissed by nature. People often ask, "Don't you get bored walking the same route all the time, always with the same scenery?" I never get bored because each day there is a different sky, which is the most beautiful scenery of all.

In addition, depending on the season, the same houses are surrounded by different scenery. They're decorated differently for various holidays and people are constantly making improvements to their homes. Once we were having a heat wave, and one family put a Christmas decoration shaped like a snowman on their lawn. The snowman made me feel cooler throughout the remainder of the walk.

For me, nothing beats walking, breathing in the fresh air, watching the sky, and being totally engrossed in my thoughts. Creative ideas are born while walking and the internal conversations are insightful. I look forward to walking throughout my whole life.

If a daily walk is your choice, you can work on your posture at the same time. While walking, keep your shoulders square and your thumbs forward. Point your thumbs where you are heading; it keeps your posture straight. Exercising gives you ease of movement, it will prevent bone loss, and allow you to age more gracefully.

If one kind of exercise doesn't excite you, try something different. Walking is a staple in my life, but at times adding other exercises into my schedule has worked well. Through the years, I have tried bike riding, bowling, jump roping, jazzercise, weight lifting, resistance-band training, yoga, floor exercises, and many different exercise DVDs. They have helped, but they are not constant. Walking is not enough at times; but at other times, it's just enough.

One client, who continually makes excuses not to exercise, said, "My doctor told me to buy a treadmill." She became angry with her doctor and insisted she didn't need one for a number of reasons. Her house was too small, so it would be in the way. Besides, a treadmill costs too much money, and so on. Agreeing with each excuse, I said, "You're correct, you don't need a treadmill, you need a sidewalk." She laughed, realizing her excuses did not matter. The doctor's message was: "Get moving!"

People say they want to turn their body fat into muscle. This is impossible! That's the same thing as saying you want to turn an orange into an apple. What you want to do is lose body fat and increase muscle mass. Two people who weigh the same can look completely different depending on their composition of body fat and muscle mass. One person looks overweight, while the other appears trim and toned because muscle is dense and body fat is not.

Let me explain this. Take a scale and weigh one pound of feathers. Now, weigh one pound of brick. The feathers represent one pound of body fat and the brick, a pound of muscle mass. The volume of feathers is greater than the brick, just as the volume of one pound of body fat is greater than one pound of muscle mass, yet each still weighs a pound. A pound of fat is about one-and-a-half times the size of a pound of chopped meat. Again, the meat represents the muscle.

Lose body fat and increase your muscle mass. Muscle will burn more calories each day and speed up your metabolic rate; excess body fat will slow down your metabolic rate—and you!

So what about you? What do you like to do? How exactly will exercise benefit you? Let's answer each one of these questions.

What About You?

First get a complete physical and know what you are capable of doing or if you have any limitations. If there are limitations, know what they are. The last thing you want to do is injure yourself. An injury can be painful, but it can also last a lifetime and stop you from doing any exercise, ever! You don't want that.

If you do have limitations, get professional advice. You might benefit from hiring a personal trainer who will teach you what is best for you. The more physically fit you become, the fewer the limitations will be. Clients who are limited to only exercising the top half of their bodies can still sit in a chair and move their arms. Soon, they feel stronger and can hold one- or two-pound bars as they move their arms. While they are doing this, they are burning calories and gaining strength. If possible, they also get into a pool and exercise in water.

If you watch television for one hour, you sit through about twenty minutes of commercials. Instead of channel surfing, get up, and move at every commercial. Those clients who have done this have great results. Not only did they burn more calories, they began to put exercise into their life.

Make a list of activities you are physically able to accomplish and enjoy doing. If you enjoy what you do, you will continue. Ask others you admire what activities they enjoy. See if their exercise habits are possible for you. Fit these activities into your day or your week. Begin today, and begin slowly. In time, you can increase the amount of time or intensity level of your exercise. Make sure your exercise is a good fit with your life. Never do more exercise than your life can handle at the time. It won't be sustainable. Smile as you exercise. It feels wonderful for the rest of the day and can empower you to continue eating well all day.

What Do You Like To Do?

Your needs may be different than those of an athlete. Your objective is to lose or manage your body weight, remain healthy, and age gracefully.

If you are like me and just want to move more, first decide what you like to do. It can be as simple as turning on the music and dancing in your living room or using a hula-hoop during television commercials. Think: "What do I enjoy, and how can I fit it into my life?" Your exercise schedule and style may change from year to year; it doesn't matter.

When I started to take walks in my early thirties, my children were too young to leave home alone, so morning was my only time to walk by myself. My plan was to wake up and have morning coffee with Chris. While the kids were still asleep, and he showered, I was able to use my time to walk.

Walking in the morning gave me more energy than the extra hour of sleep. Each day began with quality time with Chris, and then by myself. It set the tone for the rest of the day, and no matter what happened my exercise was already done. Whichever other activity happened each day with the kids, like bike riding or swimming was extra. I never considered these extras as my exercise. Today, my kids are adults, and still I walk first thing in the morning. It works best for my schedule, and it is who I am.

Make a list of everything you enjoy doing. What is possible for you today? What's possible today may be impossible tomorrow; then just choose another activity.

How Will Exercise Benefit You?

» You'll have more energy. With more energy, anything seems possible.

» Exercise will improve muscle tone. The more muscle you have, the faster you burn calories.

» You'll improve your digestion, elimination, and your body's ability to better utilize food nutrients.

» You'll relax tensions, stimulate mental processes, and induce sound sleep.

» You'll maintain a healthy body weight as you improve strength, endurance, muscle coordination, flexibility, posture, and grace of body movement.

» You'll retard the signs of aging both mentally and physically, and decrease the odds of degenerative diseases.

» You'll lower cholesterol and blood pressure, and increase your quality of life.

You can incorporate activity into your day by starting with five minutes of exercise.

Then build on it. Just move. Park far away in parking lots; use the extra steps. While food shopping, leave your cart at the end of the aisle, and walk up and down the aisle. This accomplishes two things:

» You are less prone to impulse buying.

» You are forced to take extra steps.

Stop collecting calories and start expending them. Instead of calling, texting, tweeting, or e-mailing friends, take a walk with one. Use steps in place of an elevator. Use the steps in your house as exercise equipment; make a plan to climb your steps a few times a day.

One client bought herself a hula-hoop and began to use it during television commercials. She enjoyed it and quickly realized the benefits. This excited her so much that she told her co-workers. Everyone in her entire office began to use hula-hoops in the privacy of their homes. Wellness in the workplace is contagious. Use your imagination to burn your calories.

Points to Remember

» Energy leads to more energy and more productivity.

» Start small and start immediately.

» Know your limitations.

» Long-term exercise is required and must become routine.

Find the Time

"Many of us spend half our time wishing for things we could have if we didn't spend half our time wishing."
—Alexander Woollcott
(January 19, 1887 – January 23, 1943)
American critic and commentator for The New Yorker Magazine

After the birth of my first child, Megan, my mom, who had raised five children, said, "After you have raised your children, you will look back, and all those days, months, and years will be a blur." Now those years are behind us, and Mom was right! They are a blur! Thank goodness, throughout those blurry years, while concentrating on meeting the needs of my growing family, I took the time to take care of myself. To date, I'm at a healthy weight and enjoy good health. Unlike others my age, I don't rely on any medications nor do I suffer with chronic pain from years of undue stress on my bones and joints due to excess body weight. There is no secret here and it is not a miracle; I lived what I believed.

Unfortunately, many men, women, and couples have lost sight of themselves during the blur of raising a family and enduring the stresses associated with kids, jobs, finances, and extended families. Now, later on in life, they are overweight, live in chronic pain, and rely on medications to counteract the effect of years of neglect or abuse to their own bodies.

Many people may also suffer from heart ailments, diabetes, joint pain, and lack of lust for life. These conditions might be avoided had they been cognizant of their eating patterns through the blur years. To avoid this same fate, younger couples should be mindful about their eating patterns now. Prevention is power.

In any case, it makes no difference how old you are now or what stage of life you are in now. It's not too late to change. You may feel there's a dead-end ahead, but make a U-turn.

You can always have more money, homes, jobs, friends, social gatherings, clothes, shoes, and jewelry. This list could go on and on, but you can never have more time. There is no way to manufacture more time. So here's the secret: Since you can't make more time, you have to make the most of the time you have! There is 1,440 minutes in every day. How many are spent on your welfare?

We have talked about eating and exercise. Eating well, having nutritious meals and snacks, and exercising consistently, takes time and your time is precious. Isn't there always a reason why you don't have the time to do something for you? There's the key, for *you*.

The night Megan was born, my dad leaned over my hospital bed and whispered, "Don't blink. If you blink too long, she will be lying there having a baby of her own." I knew he was thinking, "Where has the time gone?" We can all ask ourselves that question, but time doesn't stop. The questions you should be asking yourself are: "What am I doing with my time?" and "Does how I spend my time make me happy and healthy?"

Every age brings different challenges and possibilities. Everything you eat today has long-term effects. Eating is not momentary. Too often we deal with temporary moods or situations by overeating. Not one person is overweight *because they eat;* they are overweight *because they overeat.*

A client told me that when she is faced with an eating challenge, she thinks, "I have so much weight to lose, why not just eat this?" I asked her how many years she has felt this way. She stared and smiled sadly at me, "Too many?" Yes, she has exhibited this behavior too many years, and today, she is overweight with physical ailments and strains on her joints. It's time for a change!

The wife of another client called me one day. She was crying. Her husband was an extremely overweight man. She called out of desperation because she was afraid of losing her husband. His health was beginning to fail, and she feared that he was not willing to make the necessary changes to survive. He was no longer able to enjoy playing with their five young grandchildren. She confided that, due to his weight, they had not had a sexual relationship in more than ten years, and she longed for him.

Think about all the people in your life who are affected by your eating and weight challenges. If more of your time were spent wisely taking care of yourself, wouldn't you have more time and energy in your life to spend enjoying your loved ones?

I received a call from a mother asking me to work with her teenage daughter, who was beginning her junior year of high school. She was overweight, and beginning to disconnect from friends and social gatherings. The mother found her daughter hiding food in her room. Thankfully, this young, beautiful high-school student also wanted help, and we worked together during her junior and senior years.

As her last two years of high school passed, the girl felt better about herself and was able to enjoy all the memorable events that high-school students experience. She enjoyed shopping with her mother for new clothes and different styles. Although oftentimes stressful for young people, searching for colleges was empowering for her. She had the confidence in herself and her abilities to apply and to attend the college of her choice. Her mother said that preparing for her senior prom was a joy; she looked beautiful in her prom gown. Her mother said to me, "She wants shoes to match her clothes and clothes that flatter her style. This was not an easy process for her, but what a great difference it made in her high-school years."

Once you become aware of the time spent mindlessly eating, you realize that time could be spent on more productive behaviors. One client claims that when she takes the time to prepare and eat healthy nutritious foods, she feels better. The time she spends taking care of her needs is well invested in her daily routine. Another client acknowledged, since she no longer spends her day mindlessly eating, she has time to do other projects she has put off for years. Previously, this woman spent her time sitting on the couch and ate snack after snack. I call that procrastination eating, when there is something that you need to do, but you don't want to do, so first you'll eat something. Once people realize this phenomenon, they find it amazing what they can accomplish in a short amount of time. Yet another client said she likes to spend her time surrounded by upbeat, motivated people. They help her stay excited, which encourages her to use her time in a more positive manner.

Twenty-four hours a day, seven days a week, four weeks a month, twelve months a year, and how many years is anyone's guess. Pick the very same time next week, next month, or next year. Chances are you will either weigh more or weigh less. Either way, your choices have dictated the outcome.

It's all within your power. Where do you want to be? What do you have to do to make it happen? Where do you find the time?

Take an objective look at your day. Where is your time spent wisely? Where is it wasted? Take your wasted time and make good use of it, keeping in mind there is a difference between wasted time and spare time. Make a list of everything you need to accomplish today, including the time for needed sleep. When you are well rested, you will be more productive. Look at that list again. What's not necessary? Can it wait for another day when you have more time?

I received the following e-mail from a client of mine: "I did horrible yesterday. I am so frustrated with myself. All I can think of is eating unhealthy things. I have got to change my thinking. I am doing worse and worse with my decisions. I am not giving up (although looking at what I eat, you would think that I already have). Today is a new day."

My reply: "Why? Why is that all you can think of? Focus on other things. Maybe that's the issue. Is there something you don't want to think about and food is the replacement thought?" She wrote back: "That is a very good question. I may be trying to avoid my to-do list. That is definitely something for me to think about. Thanks."

Again, we call this behavior procrastination eating. How often do you have something that you should do, but don't want to do, so you eat? Is that a useful way to spend time?

Another e-mail: "Hi there. Last night, I enjoyed 3-4 glasses of wine and paid for it today. I found the article 'Weight Coming Back?' on your website. I like the idea of taking back control." It is never too late to take back control! Drinking alcohol will lower your resistance to eating. So, in her statement, I read, *"I drank and ate too much last night."* How many years do you want to spend your time uselessly and feeling the way this woman did?

Many people claim they have no time. Busy people usually know how to manage their time and be productive, while others waste time and accomplish little.

Prioritize each day. One client has two young children under five, one still in diapers. She works full time and has an hour commute to and from work. She takes care of her home, her family, and herself. She finds the time to meet with me weekly to work on her eating patterns, health, and weight loss. She has seen the health issues that her mother has to endure and believes this could also be her destiny. Part of our work together is to prioritize.

A few weeks ago, this particular client's priority was to take her kids to the park to play instead of working overtime. Could her family use the extra money? Absolutely, but she and the kids needed the playtime more. Again, time is a finite commodity, not money. Had she not taken the time to spend quality time with her children, she might have eaten mindlessly for days to overcome the guilt. Guilt is when your actions do not align with your goals. Guilt can be the most fattening emotion.

Another client was so overwhelmed with her family and work schedule that she was feeling guilty about not having enough quality time with her children. I suggested that she make appointments with her children, such as: Sunday, we'll go shopping together or Friday evening, we'll play a game together. Whatever worked in the current week, the children still looked forward to their time together and the mother no longer felt guilty. Eating due to guilt was eliminated and life became less stressful because everyone looked forward to the family time. This works if you keep your word. If you don't follow through with your planned time together, your words will have no merit. If something more important arises, you explain the new situation in detail to the kids and immediately make a new plan with them.

As they age, many people are more afraid to go to the doctor for physicals because they are afraid of getting negative results. The time you spend taking care of your nutritional needs is an investment in your future and your health. There is no better news than to get positive results at your physical. In order to hear those good reports, invest the time each day to eat healthily, exercise, and get regular physical exams.

Convenient, quick eating leads you to be overweight. Americans are the most overweight people on the planet. We are hooked on fast food, processed foods, frozen foods, and believe it or not, diet foods. Foods that are already prepared for your entire family are usually enormous, as well as have a lot of fat and sodium. In an effort to multitask and save time and energy, we eat while we are doing other things. This leads us to mindlessly eat far too much! Be honest with yourself; eating this way does not save time or energy.

In fact, eating this way steals your energy. Eating heavy fat, fast, processed, pre-prepared, convenience foods—or foods that are low in nutrients in order to be low calorie (diet foods)—will cause you to be lethargic.

Second, you decrease the number of years you live by eating these foods. Rethink how you can better spend precious minutes by preparing healthy foods and incorporating exercise in your life order to increase your years. What a wonderful trade-off! If you spend more of your minutes now to be healthy, there could be more quality years to enjoy later. That's time management at its best!

Most often it's not what we do that is so time consuming: It's how we do it. Re-evaluate the how. Find different, more efficient ways to achieve the same outcome.

A client's doctor asked her if she had ever seen an elderly person weighing what she weighs. Because this woman weighed upward of 300 pounds, her answer was no. Her doctor's retort to that was: "That's because people at your weight do not live to be elderly." Wow! That comment encouraged her to spend time to take care of her body now, so she might add years to her life expectancy.

Another client, who also weighed over 300 pounds, was desperate to change his eating, smoking, and drinking habits. He understood that he needed to this, but was not willing to put the time and effort into this change. He continually lamented, "If I don't do this, I will die." Nonetheless, he canceled our appointments and never found the time to follow through on the strategies we discussed. After a while, he stopped our appointments all together. This pattern repeated about four times. You have to believe you are worth the extra time and effort. Sadly, at age forty-nine, he suffered a fatal heart attack. "If I don't do this, I will die." Those words ring in my head. Unfortunately he was correct. Were his destructive habits fair to his two young sons? Is overeating, drinking, and smoking worth shortening your life? Nothing tastes good enough to end your life early.

On September 13, 2011, my husband Chris suffered a heart attack, followed by quintuple bypass surgery. He was fifty-seven. This was a shocking and life-altering experience for us all. Chris's surgeon said what had saved him was he wasn't overweight, didn't drink or smoke, didn't have hypertension, nor was he diabetic. We were assured that because of these facts he would come through the surgery fine and go on to live a healthy life. In hindsight, there were signs in prior months such as shortness of breath, fatigue, and tightness in his chest. Most signs he explained away to himself as indigestion or stress and never articulated to me or anyone else what he was experiencing. He was the one who called the doctor, and the doctor sent him immediately to the hospital. Thankfully, he continues to eat well, resist various foods he once ate, exercise, see his cardiologist, take his medication, watch his cholesterol, and enjoy his life. This experience was life altering, not life ending.

Sometimes people say that the time must be right to lose weight, or that they need to be ready. No, you must make the time right, and you will be ready! Clients have said that calling me to schedule that first appointment was one of the hardest phone calls to make. Some said it took months of, "I'll call her today," before they actually made the call. It is very hard to *admit*, that you need help or guidance, and equally as difficult to *ask* for guidance. How much of your time is spent procrastinating and putting off asking for help, guidance, and support? Still, during that time, procrastination eating is evident. Spend time more usefully. Make the call, ask the question, and get the help.

Here's an e-mail from a client who stopped meeting with me because, as she told me, she had too much going on in her life and no longer had time to meet:

"I never thought I would get this heavy again. Last year, four specific things happened that encouraged me to eat too much and very wrong. I don't believe in making excuses, but I can see where life got so stressed for me, I wasn't thinking of my well-being at all... I didn't have time. Forty pounds was added on like nothing. As far as how I feel, very disappointed in myself, very embarrassed in public, ugly, frustrated having a million nice things to wear and can't. I feel physically ill, because my knees are real bad now, and my hip and back have problems, too. I feel young inside, but old on the outside. Where am I, who am I? I'm not who I see in the mirror. I am still here, but covered with protective padding underneath all the layers. I hide I guess. At times I do feel sorry for myself having an eating problem. I hate it, because it shows on the outside to everyone, I can't keep it private. I have very good friends, and we talk about it all and it helps, but these are all very personal situations, and they differ from everyone else's. Life is a work in progress and unfortunately food has an important place. Of course all these feelings I have affect how I handle everything else in my life. So I'm tired."

So often, our crowded minds make us feel rushed and exhausted. Listen to all that chatter in your mind. Make a list of everything going on in your mind, and then look at the list. First, eliminate things of no importance, which allows you to make a plan and prioritize the important things. When you make a list, your tasks are listed just once. In your head, the echoes make that one item seem like 100 items.

When you eat, eat! Clear your mind, remove distractions, and think about what you are eating. This means no television, reading, shopping, driving, or anything else. Background music and light conversation are okay. Soft music can slow down your eating. Some people eat so fast they could almost make sparks with their knives and forks! Eating too fast doesn't give your mind time to register on how much you've already downed, and leads to uncontrolled eating. Food needs to nourish and satisfy your body, but at the same time, it must nourish and satisfy your mind. Your mind needs to say: "I ate, I enjoyed, and I'm done. I can move on to my next activity." If your mind is not in tune with your eating, it will never feel nourished and satisfied, leading you to overeat.

A rested person has an easier time managing his or her weight. Get enough sleep. Overtired = Overeating. Each morning, you have a new twenty-four hours to spend. Are you making the most of your day?

My daily schedule is never the same. At one time, I was a full-time mother. Now my hours belong to me. I spend them exercising, meeting with clients, attending business meetings, personal appointments, speaking engagements, phone calls, family obligations, and seeing personal friends. I want time to be with Chris, and my adult children whenever possible.

Every day I plan two things first in the morning: what I'm going to wear, and what and when I'm going to eat. I plan my meals and snacks into my day, looking at my schedule to decide what's best for me to eat and at what time I'm going to eat. It's that important. What I wear is also a key decision. When I feel good, I eat well; but if I feel sloppy, I eat sloppy. It's the body, mind, and mouth connection.

Sounds crazy? It works. I never miss a meal or a snack; that's also important. I have had clients tell me "I'm too busy to eat" or "I forgot to eat." That amazes me! I have never been too busy to eat nor have I ever forgotten to eat. You may eat at different times each day, depending on your schedule of events, but eating should still be planned. Plan your eating into each day. It takes just a few minutes each morning and will soon become a habit.

In my travels overseas, my own observation is that small European towns have vendors selling fresh fruits, vegetables, meats, fish, and bread. There are no quick processed foods. People buy their food fresh daily. Europeans rest during the day, closing down their business for a couple of hours. How do they find the time for this lifestyle, and we can't find the time to chop salad fixings? Our life is fast paced. We rush from one place to the next in an effort to "get everything done."

Women my age or older, who are losing weight usually *not* for the first time, say time and again that for years they ate what was left on their children's dinner plates as they cleaned the kitchen each night.

One client, living in the same home as her thirty-five-year-old daughter, said, "I don't understand why my daughter continually offers me the food left on her dinner plate." This client didn't make the connection that her daughter has been taught since childhood that Mom eats leftover scraps. Once Mom became aware of this dynamic, she was able to overcome eating scraps, allowing her to focus on *her* plate and *her* food. Be aware of any eating patterns before they last for thirty-five years.

Another client claims that when she has an argument with her adult daughter, all she can think of is eating. She was asked to disconnect her eating with their argument. This took time, work, and perseverance. She finally realized that she could disconnect the two, and once she accomplished this she realized she was no longer arguing with her daughter. She wondered, "Did I argue with her all these years as an excuse to eat?" We may never know.

One client of mine told me that when he dropped food on the floor he would pick it up and eat it. My immediate response was, "Like an animal?" (In that moment, I thought, "A dog eats food that falls on the floor.") I quickly said: "I'm sorry. I shouldn't have said that." He thought for a second and replied, "No, don't be sorry. That's correct, like an animal. I've never thought of it that way." He never ate scraps off the floor again. Become aware of all the useless reasons you eat.

As the years pass, our lives go through many different cycles. With each cycle, our eating must change. Think about how differently you will eat in each cycle of your life. Think about where you are now in your life. Look at your schedule each day. Where can you fit in preparing your food, and when will you eat it? However, always expect things to change, and change with them.

Find time for breakfast, the most important meal. It has been said that we should eat breakfast like a king, lunch like a queen, and dinner like a pauper. As Americans, this is not our schedule. Never start your day without breakfast. It's all right to eat the same breakfast until you tire of it. When something works, ride it as long as it works. When it stops working, find something new. Sometimes it's easy and timesaving to eat the same breakfast. Make it nutritious, and let it start you on a healthy course of eating for the day.

If you are not eating breakfast because you don't have the time, make time. Take one minute from each morning activity. Take a quicker shower, blow your hair out quicker, shave quicker, put on makeup faster, have your clothes ready beforehand, or let the kids and spouse do something on their own. You just saved a few minutes, and that's all it takes for breakfast. It doesn't have to be a big breakfast, but you need to start your metabolism. When you eat, *eat!* Even at breakfast! You don't have to have breakfast first thing in the morning. Have a glass of milk or a piece of fruit to start your metabolism. Then, when things calm down a bit, eat your breakfast. Schedule breakfast when it works best for you.

Eating a healthy breakfast gives you more energy to make you more efficient both mentally and physically in your daily activities. A few minutes spent creatively in the morning gives you more energy and time during the day.

Stay away from refined sugars at breakfast such as muffins, pastries, and bagels. Some think eating a bran muffin for breakfast is healthy. If you eat a bran muffin, call it what it really is, "A piece of cake." These foods make you feel energized for a short time, and then deprive you of your energy because of the sugar low they create. A breakfast consisting of a protein and a carbohydrate item (noted in the last chapter of the book) is a great time management tool for your day, *every* day. This combination will give you the energy and staying power you need for your morning.

Make time every day for lunch, and fit it into your schedule. Between going to office meetings and trying to accomplish work at their desks, many say they have a hard time fitting lunch in their workday. Teachers seem to have a particularly hard time scheduling lunch to coordinate with their teaching schedules. Some teachers, especially high-school teachers, have their lunch period at 9:30 in the morning. How absurd, but that's their schedule. Together, we work out an eating plan for those days. Although 9:30 AM might not seem like lunchtime, they need to eat something and save lunch until later on in the day. With a healthy lunch, you can be more productive all afternoon. Once again, this is a better use of your time.

Plan your time more efficiently while shopping in the food store. In the past, if you just walked the perimeter of the food store you would have all the food you needed such as fresh produce, milk, eggs, bread, and meat. However, grocery stores have gotten wise to this and now have placed their bakery, deli, soda, beer, diet foods, and assorted fattening impulse-buying snack foods around the perimeter. The more steps you take in the food store the more you purchase, so food stores are now mega stores. During the day, the stores play slow love songs as women shop to encourage them to think of their loved ones at home and to purchase their favorite foods. The food carts have gotten larger with the hope you won't be satisfied until you have a full cart. Bakeries are usually located by the front door. As you walk in, the wonderful aromas entice you to purchase baked goods. Coupons, double coupons, and weekly sale items create a buying frenzy. Isn't it nice that they conveniently located free food samples at the end of aisles for your tasting pleasure? No! You'll buy foods you never wanted, but will surely eat after they are in your house. You may even convince yourself that you have bought it for someone else.

The food store is a mind game and a minefield. It is critical to your weight management and your time management to carefully purchase foods in the store. Always go with a list. The few minutes it takes you to write the list saves you wasted time in the store. The list will benefit you, even if it's left home in error. Never go shopping hungry; you will give in to every urge and marketing ploy aimed at you to purchase foods you didn't need or want.

There are thousands of different food items in the store. The front of the product is designed to get you to buy. The nutrition label will be on the back or bottom of the container. It's a fair assessment that out of every hundred items in your grocery store, eighty of them are detrimental to your weight management and your health. The good news is that twenty out of every hundred will aid and encourage your health and body weight. Take the time to read labels, and be aware of everything you purchase. If you see words on labels that you can't pronounce, even on the so-called diet foods, don't buy it so you don't eat it.

Look in other people's carts to see if there is something in there you have not tried and might want to try. Ask them about the food item and where they found it. Take a few extra minutes to look for new items. The stores are full of them. With different foods on hand to prepare, you will save time during the week because the foods you like will be readily available in your home. The few extra minutes you spend in the store are worth it. The forethought has been done, the guesswork about what to eat or what to make is eliminated, and the floundering ceases. Stop running into the food store and picking the same boring items week after week, year after year, decade after decade. Find new foods to enjoy and add them to your shopping lists.

Take the time needed to plan what you eat, prepare what you plan, and then eat. Eating healthily saves time in your day and your life. When you are in control of your eating, you are in control of so many other circumstances in your life. Out-of-control eating leads to out-of-control reactions to other situations during the day. Eating left up to chance and convenience never leads to a healthy body weight. You really must take the time for yourself to think and plan your foods. In the beginning, this will seem like an overwhelming task. Nonetheless, put some work into it and give it time. If you devote the time needed, this kind of planning becomes second nature.

Another dynamic that could get in the way of better health for you is the inability to think of yourself. Do you think of everyone else first? Do your job, children, spouse, parents, and friends all come before you? When you make your needs as important as others and no one more important than the next, everyone's needs are met. This doesn't mean you are selfish or that anyone is left out. It does mean that everyone will have to learn to compromise and prioritize. This is not selfish; it's self-love.

Chris's cardiologist said: "Studies show that a married man, on average, will live longer than a single man, while a single woman will live longer than a married one." Interesting...

Have you ever thought: "Why don't I ever put myself first?" That's an unrealistic expectation and may never happen. However, you do need to make yourself as important as everyone else. In each situation, ask yourself, "Are *my* needs and *your* needs being met?" If not, compromise, negotiate, and communicate to make it happen. Soon, that will be natural for you.

Choose relationships that are worthy of you and propel you forward in every aspect of your life. Create an environment to enable you to succeed in your quest for health and wellbeing. Always be cognizant of your body, mind, and mouth connection. Your mouth will react to the thoughts in your mind, and your body will show the effects of how your mouth reacts. Be in command of your thoughts and the food that enters your mouth and you will be in command of your body.

Points to Remember

- » Spend your time surrounded by upbeat, motivated people.
- » Our crowded minds make us feel rushed.
- » You are worth the time and effort you put forth for your well-being.
- » Make you and your needs as important as your loved ones' needs are.

Now, the Science

Here's an easy guide to good nutrition to follow daily. Leave the science to the scientist and follow these healthy steps to good nutrition and a thin life.

Water helps weight loss. Are you drinking enough water? Why drink water? There are all kinds of studies on drinking water. Water is essential for digesting food and absorbing nutrients. It carries nutrients and oxygen via the bloodstream to cells and carries wastes out of the body. Water is critical in regulating body temperature and preventing constipation. You are welcome to drink other drinks as well, but make water a priority and stay away from sugary drinks. For health reasons, everyone should drink six to eight, eight-ounce glasses of water each day. The more you weigh, the more water you should have each day. Water will suppress the appetite and help the body metabolize stored fat. Drinking enough water is the best remedy for excess fluid retention. When the body gets the water it needs for survival, there is no longer a threat of dehydration; it will then release all unnecessary stored fluid. Water helps maintain proper muscle tone and helps prevent the sagging skin common in weight loss. Shrinking cells are buoyed by water;

it plumps the skin and leaves it clear, healthy, and resilient. In my opinion, water is the best face-lift. Remember these important points:

» Excess fluid shows up as excess weight.

» To release excess fluid, drink more water.

» Drinking water is essential to weight loss.

» Increase your amount of water if you are overweight, if you exercise, or if the weather is hot and dry.

» You'll know if you're drinking enough water when your urine is clear.

Proteins are found in dairy foods, eggs, fish, poultry, meats, grains, nuts, legumes, and vegetables. Protein is a compound that builds and repairs muscle tissues. Eating too much of higher-fat proteins can lead to obesity or heart disease. Meat (especially red meat) is also a great source of iron, zinc, and Vitamin B12. Sources of lean proteins include egg whites, chicken, turkey, most fish, beans, and tofu.

Fats are important to our internal organs, so we need to make sure we have a certain amount of fat in our daily diets. Fat supplies energy, helps transport and absorb fat-soluble vitamins, and allows the gallbladder to function. We do have to limit our fat intake. Each gram of fat has 9 calories while each gram of protein or carbohydrate has 4 calories. Fat has more than double the amount of calories for the same serving size of protein or carbohydrates.

Monounsaturated Fat should be the fat used most often. These fats can lower the bad LDL cholesterol and raise the good HDL cholesterol. These fats include olive oil, peanut oils, most nuts, olives, and avocados.

Saturated Fat is the type to curb the most; it can raise bad or LDL cholesterol levels, increasing the risk of heart disease. These fats are the white fat in meats, whole milk, cheese, butter, and lard.

Omega-3 Fatty Acids seem to decrease the risk of coronary-artery disease. They are found in walnuts and fatty, cold-water fish such as salmon.

Omega-3 Fatty Acids can improve the appearance and health of your skin, nails, and hair

Carbohydrates are the body's main source of energy. Many of our vitamin and mineral needs are met through carbohydrate-rich foods.

1. **Complex Carbohydrates,** when broken down, provide the body with an abundance of glucose for energy. These foods include breads, fruits, vegetables, crackers, pasta, and grains, particularly whole grains like wheat, rice, and oats.

2. **Simple Carbohydrates** are found in foods that include added fructose, sucrose, honey, and sugars. These foods add calories, but they add very few nutrients to the diet. Eat these foods sparingly.

Milk and milk products are important at any age. Their major role is to build and maintain strong bones and teeth. They are also needed for regulating the heartbeat, contracting muscles, clotting blood, and transmitting nerve impulses. Good sources of calcium are found in milk, yogurt, cheese, salmon, and sardines. Dark green leafy vegetables and broccoli are also good sources of calcium.

Fruits and vegetables provide you with much needed vitamins. To ensure a healthy eating plan, try to incorporate at least two fruits and fill up on vegetables each day. Many of the vitamins are in the skins, so wash them well and eat the skins. Try to eat fruits and vegetables close to their natural state. Since many vitamins are lost during cooking, don't overcook vegetables.

Vitamins are required in small quantities for growth, metabolism, and overall health. Check with your doctor before taking vitamins or supplements as some vitamins can counteract some medications.

Your weight, body size, activity level, and age will dictate how many of these foods you need to eat each day. Eat a variety of foods from each food group every day because each group is vital to your health, and leaving out one group leads to deprivation. We already discussed how deprivation leads to overeating, and overeating leads to weight gain.

The 10-Step WEIGH to a Healthy Body

1. Keep smiling! A smiling person has an easier time losing weight. Breathe deeply and practice moderation and patience. Always remember that the only day that matters in your weight loss/weight management process is *today*. Today, be mindful of your body, mind, and mouth connection. Focus on balance and portion size. Eliminate sugar, artificial sweeteners, and alcohol.

2. Boredom leads you to digress to eating the foods that caused you to be overweight. Make a list of all the foods you love from each food group and mix and match. Think outside the box and combine foods you have never combined before. You'll be amazed what you enjoy.

3. Include vegetables in all meals and snacks, but never eat only vegetables. Choose different foods from each food group and add vegetables everywhere.

4. If you combine a protein and a carbohydrate, meals and snacks will sustain you longer.

5. Make sure you include small amounts of fat each day and always include dairy products, or their alternatives such as soy or almond milk. Increase water intake by drinking a cup of water before you drink any other item, and drink one cup of hot water with lemon each day.

6. Eat seasonally. Enjoy all the foods that are available for the season. This insures you are eating fresh, natural foods, rather than processed foods. The added benefit is seasonal foods cost less.

7. Eat as close to the natural state of a food as possible. For example, choose foods without nutrition labels. Eat a potato in place of French fries or chips, or chicken in place of chicken sausage. Make foods with a nutrition label the exception, not the rule.

8. Include fruit each day, realizing that for some, eating fruit alone will cause you to feel hungry. Include a protein item with fruit. No one is overweight because they eat too much fruit, but too much fruit can stop a weight loss. Beware of the hand-to-mouth motion, whether it's fruit, carrots, or a calorie-laden product.

9. In order to attain and keep a healthy body weight, treat sweets, alcohol, and other foods that are not "weight-loss friendly" as special food. Use them sparingly, carefully, and in control.

10. You want to empower yourself, not deprive yourself. If you feel you have overeaten something, there is no time like the present to gain control. Go back to the step you need to practice. Don't wait until tomorrow; tomorrow never comes. The years slip away, guilt sets in, and weight returns. There is no room for guilty feelings in a successful, sustainable weight loss.

While trying to lose weight, keeping a food diary is important and monitoring portion sizes is vital. The food diary is your blueprint to your weight loss. If you are not getting the results you expect, you can always look back and investigate why. Maybe it's too much of a certain food, not enough of another. Portions may be too large or too small. Honesty with your food diary will also alleviate mindless eating. This is not something you must do forever, but do it for now.

A client of mine had kept a food diary, which had helped her to achieve a substantial weight loss. However, after she had stopped writing in the diary, she began gaining a little weight each week. I asked her to keep an honest diary for the next week, so we could examine it together. She agreed and soon realized that she had not been paying attention to what food she had been eating. Within two weeks of keeping her diary again, she lost the four pounds that had crept back. When you keep a food diary, you will not only gain insight, you will get results. The diary shows the variety of foods that you have been eating. You get different nutrients from various sources, allowing your body a more efficient weight loss.

Again, I advise eating a protein with your carbohydrate at breakfast. For your other two meals, try one focused on vegetables with some protein and a little fat, and one focused on protein with some vegetables, a carbohydrate, and a little fat. When snacking, think protein along with a fruit for snack.

Cooking Tips for Lower-Calorie Cooking

- Boiling vegetables for too long will reduce the vitamin content. Vegetables are done when they are crisp. Eat the well-cleaned skins; most of the nutrients are found in the skins.
- Cut vegetables in large pieces to prevent loss of nutrients. Some nutrients dissolve in water so do not soak vegetables.
- Use different herbs and spices and low-calorie seasonings. There are many varieties from which to choose. Keep experimenting! Try a new seasoning each week.
- Broiling, roasting on a rack, or grilling are smart methods of cooking meat, which allow the fat to drip away from the meat that you will eat.
- When broiling, don't baste with oils, butter, or margarine.
- When making gravy, cool the liquid first, and skim the fat collected on top.

- Boiling and stewing are effective cooking methods for less tender cuts of meat. Trim all visible fat from the meat, and if boiling, discard all liquid. With stews, allow stew to cool, and remove all fat that has hardened on top before warming and serving stew.

- The leanest cuts of meat are the loin, round, and leg. Loin chop, London broil, top round, sirloin tip roast, tenderloin, arm pot roast, bottom round, boneless sirloin steak, strip steak, and filet mignon are examples of lean cuts.

- *Sit down* to a nice meal. Presentation is everything.

Let's Go Out to Eat

- Eat before you go. (This is to control your appetite, not suppress it.)
- Check websites for menus, call ahead to see what will be served if you are attending a planned party, and know what you want to eat before you go.
- Suggest a restaurant where you know the menu. If possible, you pick the restaurant.
- You'll pay a high cost in calories eating the free extras such as bread, Chinese noodles, and nacho chips.
- Order a big glass of water, and be sure to drink it.
- Go easy on alcoholic beverages. They contain a high amount of empty calories and can change your mood, which may cause you to overeat.
- When you are at a social gathering and food is abundant,

remember to socialize. Less eating is done when more socializing takes place.

» Avoid ordering foods that are described on the menu with the following words: breaded, béarnaise, au gratin, Parmesan, cream, hollandaise, crispy, fried, flaky, or escalloped.

» Order foods described with these words: roasted, grilled, broiled, poached, stir-fried, or steamed. Stick to sauces that are stock-based or red.

» Choose a-la-carte items, and avoid all-you-can-eat menus.

» Always be aware of portion sizes. You can ask your server for the exact serving size for any item on the menu. If they do not know, they can find out from the kitchen. Your serving is the restaurant's inventory; they know the amount of food on your plate!

» Take half of your meal home to enjoy another day.

» Order a salad and two appetizers for your meal. Truly have it your way.

» Socializing is vital to our well-being.

EAT, SOCIALIZE, LAUGH, AND LIVE!

Epilogue

Through experience and research, Margaret Marshall has developed an innovative way of reaching out to people and teaching them how to get and keep in shape. She shows you the simplicity of implementing these thoughts and techniques into your lifestyle, as well as how to make these habits last throughout the stages of your life. She believes that caring for your body is a lifetime mission that can give you a competitive edge in your personal and professional life.

Margaret Marshall is a nationally recognized speaker, who addresses a variety of topics regarding health and wellness through weight control. With more than a quarter of a century of experience, she is a recognized expert in her field and has worked personally with nearly 10,000 individuals. She has also done extensive work in workplace wellness issues and frequently speaks to corporations and organizations.

Margaret Marshall is president of Margaret Marshall Assoc., Inc., and the founder of the "Why Weight" Coaching Method. She is a member of the National Speakers Association and serves on the board of the New York

City Chapter. She has been featured on television and radio, as well as magazines and newspapers.

Margaret lives on Long Island, New York, with her husband Chris. After raising their two children, Megan and Michael, the couple has entered the so-called empty-nest stage of their life. However, Margaret and Chris consider it a return to the honeymoon stage!

For further information about how to arrange a media interview with Margaret Marshall, hire her to speak at your next business event, or make an appointment for personal coaching, please visit: www.MargaretMarshallAssoc.com.

You can also follow Margaret Marshall on Facebook and LinkedIn.

33392056R00068

Made in the USA
Lexington, KY
23 June 2014